35

Leg Pain

W9-CYU-271

Leg Pain

Magruder C. Donaldson, MD

Chairman of Surgery,
MetroWest Medical Center
Framingham and Natick, Massachusetts
Associate Professor of Surgery
Harvard Medical School
Division of Vascular Surgery
Brigham and Women's Hospital
Boston, Massachusetts

Blackwell
Futura

Blackwell Publishing, Inc., 350 Main Street, Malden, Massachusetts 02148-5020, USA
Blackwell Publishing Ltd, 9600 Garsington Road, Oxford OX4 2DQ, UK
Blackwell Publishing Asia Pty Ltd, 550 Swanston Street, Carlton, Victoria 3053, Australia

04 05 06 07 5 4 3 2 1

Donaldson, Magruder C.
 Leg pain / Magruder C. Donaldson.
   p. ; cm.
 Includes bibliographical references and index.
 ISBN 1-4051-1645-5
 1. Leg—Diseases—Diagnosis. 2. Leg—Pathophysiology. 3. Pain.
 [DNLM: 1. Leg—pathology. 2. Leg—physiopathology. 3. Pain—etiology. 4. Pain—
therapy. WE 850 D676L 2004] I. Title.
 RC951.D66   2004
 617.5'807—dc22

                                                                   2004000501

A catalogue record for this title is available from the British Library

Acquisitions: Steven Korn
Production: Julie Elliott
Typesetter: Graphicraft Limited, Hong Kong, in 9.5/12pt Palatino
Printed and bound in India by Replika Press Pvt. Ltd., Kundli 131 028

For further information on Blackwell Publishing, visit our website:
www.blackwellfutura.com
www.blackwellpublishing.com

Notice: The indications and dosages of all drugs in this book have been recommended in the medical literature and conform to the practices of the general community. The medications described do not necessarily have specific approval by the Food and Drug Administration for use in the diseases and dosages for which they are recommended. The package insert for each drug should be consulted for use and dosage as approved by the FDA. Because standards for usage change, it is advisable to keep abreast of revised recommendations, particularly those concerning new drugs.

Contents

List of contributors

Sang Cheol Bae, MD
Associate Professor of Medicine, Head; Division
of Rheumatology, Head; Section for Clinical
Epidemiology and Economics, The Hospital for
Rheumatic Diseases, Hanyang University College
of Medicine, Seoul, Korea

Magruder C. Donaldson, MD
Chairman of Surgery, MetroWest Medical Center,
Framingham and Natick, MA; Associate Professor
of Surgery, Harvard Medical School; Division
of Vascular Surgery, Brigham & Women's
Hospital, Boston, MA

Matthew H. Liang, MD
Professor of Medicine, Harvard Medical School,
Brigham & Women's Hospital, Boston, MA

Tamara L. Martin, MD
Assistant Professor of Orthopedic Surgery,
Harvard Medical School, Department of
Orthopedics, Brigham & Women's Hospital,
Boston, MA

Scott D. Martin, MD
Assistant Professor of Orthopedic Surgery,
Harvard Medical School, Department of
Orthopedics, Brigham & Women's Hospital,
Boston, MA

Srdjan S. Nedeljković, MD
Assistant Professor of Anesthesia, Department of
Anesthesia, Harvard Medical School, Director of
Resident Education, Pain Management Center,
Brigham & Women's Hospital, Boston, MA

David C. Preston, MD
Director, Neuromuscular Service, University
Hospitals of Cleveland; Professor of Neurology,
Case Western Reserve University, Cleveland, OH

Foreword

This small volume is devoted to one of the commonest patient complaints encountered by practitioners of adult medicine, and one which frequently presents the initial examining physician with a diagnostic conundrum. Few primary care physicians, emergency room physicians, or for that matter, medical or surgical subspecialists are thoroughly familiar with the neurologic, orthopedic, immunologic, and vascular causes of leg pain. Moreover, help from the medical literature requires access to multiple texts from diverse medical and surgical specialties.

Leg Pain should go a long way towards solving this dilemma since it brings together, in a compact and easily transportable volume, expertise from the fields of vascular surgery, neurology, orthopedics, and rheumatology, to offer insights into the clinical signs and symptoms associated with leg pain of diverse origins. As a practical point, many of the authors of the eight chapters in the volume have emphasized distinguishing features of the various types of leg pain, which can be determined by a simple history and physical examination. Most chapters also include data in tabular form, which can greatly aid in arriving at a correct diagnosis.

This compact volume I believe will be particularly useful for medical students, medical and surgical house officers, primary care physicians and emergency room physicians. It should make the next encounter with a patient complaining of leg pain a good deal less perplexing.

John A. Mannick, MD

Acknowledgments

The editor would like to gratefully acknowledge the support and expertise of the contributing co-authors, particularly their willingness to work towards a relatively uniform format and style necessary to fit the goal of a concise and general handbook. Review of some sections by outside readers is greatly appreciated, including especially Peter McL. Black, MD and Michael Wilson, MD. In addition, thanks are due to the multidisciplinary faculty of a symposium on leg pain organized by the editor and conducted at the University of Connecticut School of Medicine years ago. The encouragement of one participant in particular, Dr Frank Davidoff, helped create the impetus to proceed with a basic textbook on a common subject which all too often seems to fall into the cracks between our subspecialties. Finally, I am most thankful for the steadfast devotion of our publisher, Steven E. Korn, for his encouragement and wise advice over the course of putting this book together.

CHAPTER 1

Overview

Magruder C. Donaldson

Everyone experiences pain and discomfort in the lower extremities at frequent intervals. Bruises and sprains as well as general leg fatigue are completely typical of our bipedal existence, and we rely on sensory signals from the leg to alert us to the need for care and rest. Self-limited and essentially physiological leg discomfort occasionally becomes a chronic disabling complaint, however, precipitating medical consultation.

A careful history and physical examination most often reveal the explanation for leg pain and lead to an expedient, satisfactory solution. However, all too frequently multiple chronic conditions coexist with overlapping and confusing symptom complexes. In some instances, there may be clear objective findings compatible with two or more explanations for the patient's complaints, making it difficult to choose the proper therapy.

Case study

Mr O'Leary is a 67-year-old retired diabetic construction worker with a 50-year history of smoking, longstanding hypertension controlled on a regimen including a β-blocker and a diuretic, a history of left leg deep vein thrombosis at age 42 with subsequent secondary varicose veins and mild stasis dermatitis, bilateral hip and knee arthritis and a history of work-related back injury at age 61. He presents with left leg symptoms consisting of fatigue and heaviness upon arising in the morning, pain in the knee and calf with exercise, and pins and needles with cramping in the foot at night. He is no longer able to keep up with his dog on his habitual walk in the park, and in recent weeks has had difficulty sleeping.

Mr O'Leary is typical of many patients who limp into the healthcare system having been sidelined from work or leisure activities by loss of their means of locomotion. In his case, pain has progressed to a point where it is starting to interfere with sleep, one of the body's truly vital functions. Otherwise appearing healthy, Mr O'Leary is tired out and anxious not only to relieve the pain but to be sure that he is not about to develop gangrene or a blood clot in the lung and that he is not harboring some other dreaded threat to life or limb.

The healthcare team, often initially represented by a nurse or physician in an emergency room, walk-in clinic or general medical office, is faced with a relatively complicated history to sift for diagnostic hints. An array of diagnostic tests is available, many of which would involve significant expense, some measure of discomfort and risk, consultation with one or more specialists and much inconvenience for the relatively immobile patient. The main goal of the initial encounter should be to secure a working diagnosis with plans for early referral for confirmation of the diagnosis by testing or consultation where appropriate. No less important should be provision of some measure of reassurance and explanation to the patient in combination with the means for at least temporary pain management.

The most important early diagnostic step is a careful history. It will almost always allow preliminary differentiation between urgent and more elective situations and between a condition localized to the leg itself and one more probably related to systemic illness. The pain's location, character, temporal pattern and relationship to various positions and activities are particularly revealing. The presence of concurrent illness, antecedent injury and medications will provide clues. Past illness, occupational history and risk factors for chronic conditions should be elicited. Finally, details such as a history of intolerance to analgesics, anti-inflammatory agents or radiographic contrast may influence early diagnostic or therapeutic plans.

Examination of the lower extremities will test the working hypothesis developed during the patient interview, but other important evidence may be found in the general physical. Atherosclerosis and arthritis affect many parts of the body, and a full review of blood pressure, peripheral pulses, bruits, abdominal pulsations, joints and back is fundamental. Diabetes, alcoholic neuropathy, tabes dorsalis and gout are other examples of systemic illnesses with multiple physical findings in addition to those in the leg. Specific maneuvers during the lower extremity examination may be pathognomonic, with no need for extensive supportive laboratory testing.

Radiological, non-invasive vascular or other laboratory evaluation should be aimed at clarifying the diagnosis when it is still unclear after a careful history and physical. Use of the laboratory is most helpful when more than one entity is present, as in Mr O'Leary's case. In some circumstances, even when the diagnosis is obvious, objective measures are useful to quantify the abnormality and to allow comparison with later study after one or another form of management. This rationale would be appropriate, for example, for study of a patient with chronic arterial disease. An underlying priority, of course, is to direct investigation in such a way as to minimize inconvenience, risk, and cost to the patient.

Early therapeutic interaction with the patient should consist of simple discussion of the likely diagnostic alternatives. This step in itself will usually provide relief of anxiety and concern about the unknown, with significant therapeutic spin-off. Most often, more specific advice will also be appropriate based on the working generic diagnosis, even before more rigorous laboratory or radiological confirmation. Thus rest, exercise, specific medications or analgesics can be prescribed to provide at least short-term relief. Definitive therapy may in fact be possible at the outset in some circumstances. Finally, appropriate and timely referral for further testing or consultation should be arranged, together with early follow-up and continuity with the initial physician when indicated.

CHAPTER 2

Pathophysiology of leg pain

Srdjan S. Nedeljković

Sensory perception depends on both reception and interpretation of information and is in part a subjective process which varies with an individual's experience. Specialized somatic sensory receptors detect the quality of normal sensory information, differentiating between light touch, stretch or pressure, vibration, change in position and pain. For each type of stimulus, the quantity of sensory input is proportional to the frequency of the afferent signals transmitted from the receptor along afferent pathways, and depends on modulation by central nervous system (CNS, spinal cord and brain) mechanisms.

In the lower extremity, sensory receptors occur in higher concentrations at anatomic boundaries such as the skin, deep fascia, periosteum and joint linings (but not cartilage). Receptors are also present in tendons, muscle, and connective tissue between muscle fibers and within blood vessel walls.

Fundamentals

Pain processing depends on transmission of noxious stimulii (mechanical, thermal, and chemical irritants) via peripheral sensory nerves. This afferent input creates an electrical impulse which reaches a threshold for encoding the stimulus and insuring propagation into the CNS (Figure 2.1). Chemical mediators may sensitize nociceptor endings and lower the threshold for response. In general, nociceptor stimulation implies the presence of noxious input sufficiently strong to represent potential danger or harm to the individual. The phenomenon of 'itch' is also signaled via these receptors, perhaps channeled centrally to differentiate from pain. Both myelinated rapid conduction (Aδ) and unmyelinated slow conduction fibers (C) are involved. The former typically serve the skin and transmit focused, sharp pain and the latter serve the deeper tissues carrying sensations of dull, poorly localized pain and temperature. In addition, there is evidence that stimulation of abnormally sensitized large fiber mechanoreceptors (Aβ) may also result in nociception (Figure 2.2).

Repeated or constant stimulation of nociceptors by tissue injury produces a sensitization phenomenon. Under such circumstances the threshold for receptor stimulation is lowered so that minimal stimulation such as light stroking of the skin produces pain at both the injured site and the surrounding uninjured tissue. Hyperalgesia is defined as an accentuated painful response

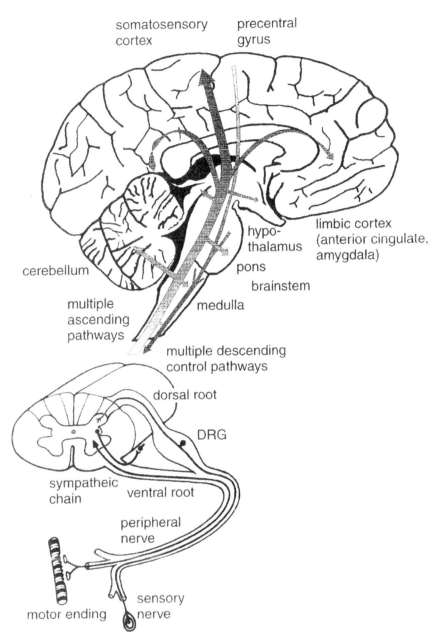

somatosensory cortex

precentral gyrus

limbic cortex (anterior cingulate, amygdala)

hypo-thalamus

pons

brainstem

cerebellum

medulla

multiple ascending pathways

multiple descending control pathways

dorsal root

DRG

sympatheic chain

ventral root

peripheral nerve

motor ending

sensory nerve

Figure 2.1 Nociceptor pathways. Afferent peripheral input creates an electrical impulse which propagates into the spinal cord and brain. Descending inhibitory pathways modulate the pain response. Reprinted with permission from Devor M. Neurobiology of normal and pathophysiological pain. In: Aronoff GM, ed. *Evaluation and Treatment of Chronic Pain,* 3rd edn. Baltimore: Williams & Wilkins, copyright 1999; 12.

Primary afferent axons

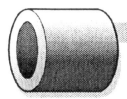

Aα and Aβ fibers

Myelinated
Large diameter
Proprioception, light touch

Aδ fiber

Lightly myelinated
Medium diameter
Nociception
(mechanical, thermal, chemical)

C fiber

Unmyelinated
Small diameter
Innocuous temperature, itch
Nociception
(mechanical, thermal, chemical)

Figure 2.2 Nociceptor types. Different pain perceptions are detected by three primary types of nociceptors. These are the small (Aδ) and large (Aβ, Aα) diameter myelinated fibers and small diameter (C) unmyelinated fibers. Adapted with permission from *Nature* and the authors (Julius D, Basbaum AI. Molecular mechanisms of nociception. *Nature* 2001; **413**:203–210) copyright 2001, Macmillan Publishers Ltd.

from a normally noxious stimulus whereas allodynia is defined as a perception of pain from a normally non-painful stimulus.

Sensory stimulation results in a spectrum of response which eventually leads to nociception. Mild mechanical aberrations may be interpreted as transient, variable or constant pressure, tightness, or pain. With increasing afferent

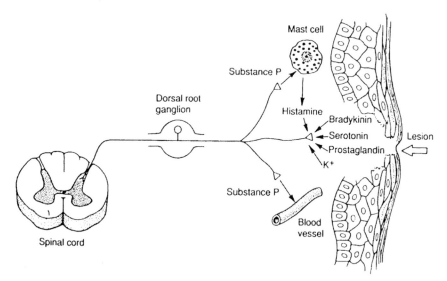

Figure 2.3 Chemical sensitizers. Inflammatory mediators are released at the site of injury, creating a sensitizing 'soup' which lowers stimulation thresholds of nociceptors. Adapted with permission from Basbaum AJ, Jessell TM. The perception of pain. In: Kandel ER, Schwartz JH, Jessell TM, eds. *Principles of Neural Science*, 4th edn. New York: McGraw-Hill, 2000; 481, with permission of the McGraw-Hill Companies.

barrage, sensory input increases until the sensory receptors reach a nociceptive threshold which is transmitted to first-order central neurons of the spinal cord gray matter and to the dorsal columns. Chemical modulators present in inflammation or after tissue injury enhance pain perception by reducing the stimulation threshold of nociceptors (Figure 2.3). Ascending pathways of nociception are then modulated by descending inhibitory controls and ultimately integrated into the somatosensory cerebral cortex, resulting in conscious pain perception (Figure 2.1). In the lower extremities, reduced nutritive blood supply to tissues can cause immediate pain at an early stage which progresses to sensory impairment and finally anesthesia as ischemia persists. Motor nerves and muscles exposed to profound ischemia also become dysfunctional but are relatively tolerant compared with sensory nerves.

In addition to afferent input involving sensory receptors, pain may be produced by direct mechanical compression of a peripheral nerve or nerve root. In the case of the lower extremity, the site of compression is frequently above the inguinal ligament, although the pain radiates along the course of the nerve in the leg itself. Other neuropathic symptoms may be caused by diseases particular to the nerves themselves or by systemic illnesses with associated neuropathological changes.

Ultimately, chronic painful stimuli may initiate a series of complicated interconnections and responses within the spinal cord and brain, producing histopathological and physiological changes in the CNS. These CNS abberations can then themselves cause a persistence of pain, even when the original afferent stimulus is no longer causing nociception. This is thought to be the basis of centrally mediated chronic pain syndromes such as deafferentiation pain, spinal cord injury pain, and phantom pain. Finally, pain has effects on cognition and affect (anxiety and fear), autonomic function (reflex vasoconstriction, pupillary dilatation, tachycardia) and involuntary motor function (reflex withdrawal, muscle cramping adjacent to injury).

Mechanical stimulation

Mechanical distortion of normal tissue anatomy produces stimulation of a variety of sensory receptors located throughout the lower extremity. External stimuli are sensed at the skin level. Pacinian corpuscles in the subcutaneous tissue detect pressure. Merkel's cells and tactile disks in the subepidermal region gauge pressure intensity. Meissner's corpuscles and hair follicle receptors in the dermis detect motion of hair or skin. Ruffini endings in the dermis detect skin stretch. All of these receptors transmit afferent signals via myelinated fast fibers. More sparsely distributed mechanoreceptors conduct sensations of tickling or crawling via unmyelinated slow fibers. Internal stimuli are sensed by receptors in joints, muscles and tendons. Pacinian corpuscles or free nerve endings in the joints, muscle spindles, and tendons are responsible for proprioception, which allows determination of position, movement and force.

Thermal and mechanical nociceptors are distributed at the skin level. Noxious mechanical insults such as pinching, compression, and sprains stimulate mechanical nociceptors in the subcutaneous and deeper tissues. When tissues are traumatized by mechanical forces, inflammatory mediators are released which greatly magnify receptor sensitivity and result in heightened pain perception.

Inflammation

Inflammation accompanies a variety of insults including mechanical trauma, infection, intravascular thrombosis, tissue infarction, and autoimmune or allergic phenomena. Numerous substances are released after these insults which mediate or facilitate the inflammatory process. These substances include histamine, serotonin, bradykinin, substance P, platelet activating factor, free radicals, tumor necrosis factor, prostaglandins, thromboxanes and leukotrienes (Figure 2.3). Histamine is released from mast cells immediately following injury and results in local vasodilatation with increased local blood flow (rubor, calor). Increased flow and capillary permeability as well as release of intracellular contents by tissue injury contribute to swelling (tumor). Pain (dolor) is produced by a combination of nociceptor stimulation related to the inciting injury, stretching of tissues due to swelling, and a lowering of nociceptive thresholds induced by inflammatory mediators and resulting in hyperalgesia and allodynia.

Sensitivity of nociceptors in peripheral tissues is increased especially by bradykinin, histamine, prostaglandins, cytokines, and by tumor necrosis factor. Prostaglandins and leukotrienes are arachidonic acid metabolites which work synergistically via vasoactive amines/kinins and leukocytes, respectively, to amplify pain. Cyclo-oxygenase inhibitors such as ibuprofen decrease pain by decreasing production of these metabolites, as well as via central mechanisms. Though the release of inflammatory mediators is essential to eventual healing, the inflammatory process itself may compound injury and result in persistent pain states in some instances.

Ischemia

Decreased oxygen delivery to tissues results in localized acidosis. Persistence of hypoxia results in cellular injury with release of intracellular products such as potassium and production of oxygen free radicals. An inflammatory response occurs with involvement of the mediators mentioned above (Figure 2.4). All of these byproducts of ischemia stimulate nociceptors. In syndromes involving reversible ischemia such as intermittent claudication, clearance of noxious byproducts by resumption of normal circulation results in diminution of pain. With prolonged ischemia, afferent nerves themselves suffer permanent ischemic damage and this may result in a chronic neuropathic pain state. Motor nerves and muscles tend to be more resistant than sensory nerves to the effects of prolonged ischemia.

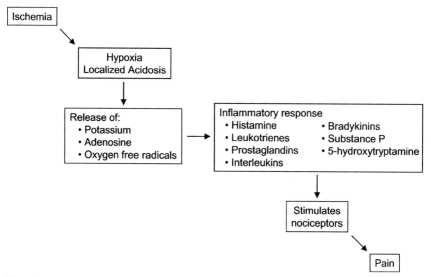

Figure 2.4 Ischemic–inflammatory pain cascade. Vascular ischemia in peripheral vascular disease can lead to hypoxia and acidosis of tissue, releasing inflammatory mediators which stimulate nociceptors. This cascade results in pain.

Neuropathy

Neuropathic pain results from increased peripheral and central sensitization, which may abnormally persist even after afferent impulses originating in the nerves themselves eventually diminish. This occurs because of (i) abnormally lowered pain thresholds due to increased sensitivity of the nervous system, (ii) increased ectopic discharge related to peripheral nerve injury, compression or disease, and (iii) increased afferent convergence which is accompanied by dysfunctional central modulation. The net result may be a 'centralization' of pain, with CNS changes which result in chronic pain which is independent of peripheral input.

In the case of blunt nerve trauma, injury over the trunk of the nerve usually creates a brief discharge with subsequent near-total loss of afferent and efferent traffic, including pain. Often, the loss of peripheral afferent input from either trauma to the nerve receptor or sharp partial or complete nerve transection results in hyperexcitability of the severed nerve endings. In these cases, ectopic afferent signals are generated by a variety of stimuli such as mechanical, thermal, ischemic and chemical (such as tissue acidosis, histamine, bradykinins, 5-hydroxytryptamine, prostaglandins, cytokines, neutrophils, etc.) (Figure 2.5). Spontaneous firing with little or no ongoing stimulus is also typical of chronic neuropathic pain. As regeneration occurs after injury, free nerve endings create ectopic hyperexcitability (i.e. neuromas), which is thought to result from the proliferation of excess voltage-sensitive sodium channels in the damaged nerve remnant. The absence of myelin in an injured nerve and the upregulation of sodium channel synthesis which results from an injury lead to enhanced neuropathic sensitivity which may become chronic if the nerve endings fail to reconnect distally.

Many diseases are associated with nerve degeneration with accompanying cycles of demyelination and regeneration. This activity leads to abnormal spontaneous discharging of the nerve, which is interpreted as a mixed array of unpleasant afferent sensations. In addition, coupling between the sensory afferent system and the sympathetic nervous system may occur, a phenomenon which is thought to contribute to allodynia and ongoing pain after nerve injury (see Figure 2.5). In sympathetically maintained pain states, such as some cases of reflex sympathetic dystrophy (RSD, now called CRPS, type 1 'complex regional pain syndrome'), pain may be relieved by sympathetic blockade. Injured afferent neurons may exhibit upregulation of adrenoreceptors, with increased α_2 adrenoreceptor release of norepinephrine, all of which may exacerbate pain.

Central modulation and plasticity

Permanent integration of pain into the CNS involves the complex interface between perception and transduction of peripheral stimuli into the CNS along with processing and modulation of stimuli and perception. Chronic noxious

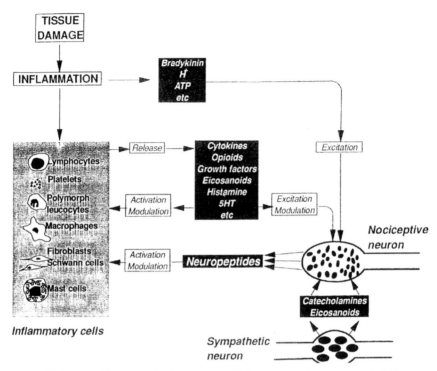

Figure 2.5 Neuropathic pain mechanisms. Injury and inflammation releases various factors that can act on nociceptive neurons and interact with the sympathetic nervous system. With permission from Rang HP, Bevan S, Dray A. Nociceptive peripheral neurons: cellular properties. In: Wall PD, Melzack R, eds. *Textbook of Pain*, 3rd edn. Copyright 1994, p. 58, with permission from Elsevier.

mechanical, inflammatory, ischemic or neuropathic sensory input initiates a series of events within the CNS with the result that perception of pain persists either out of proportion to the stimulus or in the absence of the original stimulus.

Noxious stimulation results in a hyperexcitable state in dorsal horn neurons which manifests itself by the development of 'windup', by enhancement of cutaneous receptive fields, and by the nociceptive neuron's acquisition of wide-dynamic-range (WDR) neuron properties. Windup describes a progressively increased response which occurs when nociceptive fibers are stimulated. As the nociceptive neuron acquires WDR neuron characteristics, it begins to respond even to innocuous stimuli. Activation of WDR neurons involves release of glutamate, an excitatory neurotransmitter, which stimulates the N-methyl-D-aspartate receptor, sustaining a hypersensitized state.

Chronically painful conditions such as phantom limb pain, complex regional pain syndrome, and persistent lumbar radiculopathy involve a complex interplay between the mechanisms of peripheral and central sensitization.

Amputation involves the severing of sensory and motor axons, which leads to abnormal, ectopic impulse discharge, stimulating spinal sensory pathways and triggering central sensitization. Increased sympathetic efferent activity will often exacerbate phantom pain. The fact that phantom pain can persist in spite of dorsal rhizotomy or spinal cord transection illustrates a probable central component of pain. In addition, the 'memory' that patients have of painful ulcers and other lesions on amputated extremities suggests centralization of pain. Habitual perception of pain and other sensory stimuli continues for a variable time despite the absence of the limb.

Complex regional pain syndrome is an example in which a relatively small initial stimulus in the form of trauma may result in a chronic pain syndrome which may progress to disuse atrophy and disability despite apparent healing at the site of the trauma. Sympathetic stimulation and relief of pain by sympathetic blockade in some cases suggests that sympathetic efferents may be coupled to nociceptive afferents (Figure 2.5). It has been shown that nerve injury causes sprouting of sympathetic endings in the dorsal root ganglion (DRG), thereby stimulating discharge from the DRG. Finally, in chronic lumbar radiculopathy, an initial disc herniation may lead to a release of inflammatory mediators or to actual compression, both of which may cause neuronal damage and ectopic discharge. The DRG may be compressed directly or be pulled by a herniated disc, and this may cause further ectopic neuronal discharge, possibly leading to central sensitization of pain.

Summary

In summary, sensory pain perception involves a complex interplay of afferent nociceptive pathway stimulation, impulse modulation, and peripheral and central sensitization (Figure 2.6). Mechanical stimulation and ischemia may cause release of inflammatory mediators, which results in neuronal damage and sensitization. Neuropathic pain mechanisms depend on peripheral afferent input, spontaneous ectopic discharge, and integration of pain into the CNS. Sensory coupling may occur with the sympathetic nervous system. The phenomenon of windup may occur, along with an expansion of receptive fields and the perception of non-noxious stimuli as painful.

Suggested reading

Bridges D, Thompson SWN, Rice ASL. Mechanisms of neuropathic pain. *Br J Anaes* 2001; **87**:12–26.

Codere TJ, Katz J, Vaccarino AL, Melzack R. Contribution of central neuroplasticity to pathological pain: review of clinical and experimental evidence. *Pain* 1993; **52**:259–285.

Devor M. Pain mechanisms. *Neuroscientist* 1996; **2**:233–244.

Devor M. Neurobiology of normal and pathophysiological pain. In: Aronoff GM, ed. *Evaluation and Treatment of Chronic Pain*, 3rd edn. Baltimore: Williams & Wilkins, 1999; 11–25.

I. Pain Transmission to the Spinal Cord

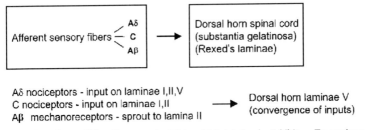

Aδ nociceptors - input on laminae I,II,V
C nociceptors - input on laminae I,II → Dorsal horn laminae V
Aβ mechanoreceptors - sprout to lamina II (convergence of inputs)

II. Activation of Dorsal Horn Receptors by EAA and Modulation by Inhibitory Transmitters

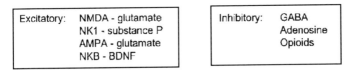

III. Pain Pathways: Spinal Cord to Brain

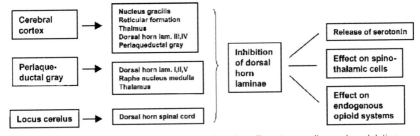

IV. Descending Modulating Pathways

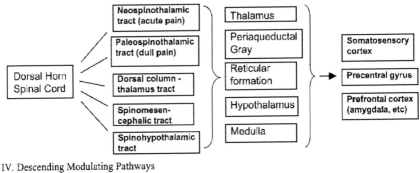

Figure 2.6 Summary of pain mechanisms demonstrating afferent ascending and modulating descending pathways.

Jensen TS. Mechanisms of neuropathic pain. In: Campbell JN, ed. *Pain—An Updated Review.* Seattle: IASP Press, 1996; 77–86.

Julius D, Basbaum AI. Molecular mechanisms of nociception. *Nature* 2001; **413**:203–210.

Kandel ER, Schwartz JH, Jessell TM. *Principles of Neural Science,* 4th edn. New York: McGraw-Hill, Inc., 2000.

Katz J, Melzack R. Pain "memories" in phantom limbs: review and clinical observations. *Pain* 1990; **43**:319–336.

Levine J, Taiwo Y. Inflammatory pain. In: Wall PD, Melzack R, eds. *Textbook of Pain,* 3rd edn. Edinburgh: Churchill Livingstone, 1994; 45–56.

McLachlan EM, Janig W, Devor M, Michaelis M. Peripheral nerve injury triggers noradrenergic sprouting within dorsal root ganglia. *Nature* 1993; **363**:543–546.

Meyer RA, Campbell JN, Raja SN. Peripheral neural mechanisms of nociception. In: Wall PD, Melzack R, eds. *Textbook of Pain,* 3rd edn. Edinburgh: Churchill Livingstone, 1994; 13–44.

Newshaw DJ, Edwards RHT, Mills KR. Skeletal muscle pain, In: Wall PD, Melzack R, eds. *Textbook of Pain,* 3rd edn. Edinburgh: Churchill Livingstone, 1994; 423–440.

Rang HP, Bevan S, Dray A. Peripheral neuropathies. In: Wall PD, Melzack R, eds. *Textbook of Pain,* 3rd edn. Edinburgh: Churchill Livingstone, 1994; 57–78.

Scadding JW. Peripheral neuropathies. In: Wall PD, Melzack R, eds. *Textbook of Pain,* 3rd edn. Edinburgh: Churchill Livingstone, 1994; 667–683.

CHAPTER 3

The initial encounter

Magruder C. Donaldson

The initial encounter with the patient suffering from leg pain is a critical depar-
ture point. The physician must develop a diagnostic impression by working
through the history and physical findings in a systematic fashion. In the process he must reach a conclusion about the level of severity and danger to life
and limb that is present and judge whether or not the patient requires expedi-
tious referral, definitive testing or direct therapy. During the interview and
exam differential diagnosis must of necessity be the foremost concern guiding
questioning and probing, but with simultaneous assessment of the impact of
the more generic issues of pain, functional disability, and danger as the evaluation proceeds. As the disease process becomes clearer, a series of thresholds
for diagnostic referrals or therapeutic action will be approached, with decisions
at each turn. This diagnostic analysis and emergence of a problem-orientated
plan are the essence of the initial assessment.

History

Questioning of the patient begins with a series of inquiries which results in a
description of the duration, pattern, quality, and character of the pain syndrome. Concurrent and past illnesses should be documented. Appropriate
details of occupational and daily activity should be established to illuminate
the true functional impact of the leg pain. A complete history should result in a
nearly diagnostic picture, leaving the physical examination and laboratory
analysis to validate and prioritize a short list of diagnostic options developed
on the basis of the patient's story. The general line of questioning should
follow the elements outlined in Table 3.1, emphasizing the differential points
noted.

Severity is inferred from the duration, intensity, and constancy of the pain,
all of which translate into some degree of functional impairment not only with
ambulation but in severe cases with other aspects of function such as social life,
emotional health, and sleep. Most times, the presence of danger is inferred
from the initial history, brief as it may be on occasions when there is an air
of urgency. For example, a frantic telephone call describing abrupt onset
of a painful cold foot in a patient who recently had undergone peripheral
arterial bypass surgery would clearly be placed at top priority. A more subtle
element of danger may be introduced when pain or pain medications disturb

Table 3.1 Historical features of leg pain.

	Mechanical	Inflammatory	Vascular		Neuropathic	
			Arterial	Venous	Root	Nerve
Character						
Cramp				X		
Ache	X	X	X			
Burn						X
Shoot					X	
Stab	X	X				
Pins and needles					X	X
Numb					X	X
Heavy			X	X		
Tired/weak			X		X	
Location						
Joint	X	X				
Muscle	X		X			
Bone	X					
Skin		X			X	X
Dermatome					X	
Distal predominance			X			X
Temporality						
Intermittent						
Worse with:						
Lying flat			X			
Straight leg raising					X	
Dependency				X		
Immobility		X				
Bending joint	X	X				
Cough					X	
Contact						X
Weight bearing	X	X				
Walking	X	X	X		X	
Better with:						
Recumbency	X					
Elevation				X		
Dependency			X			
Mobility		X				
Stand after walk			X			
Sit after walk			X		X	
Spontaneous pattern						X
Constant		X	X			X

fundamental functions like eating and sleeping. For example, an elderly frail patient with sciatica preventing sleep and requiring narcotic analgesics to the point of nausea and somnolence may be in a precarious position.

Detailed description of the pain pattern and character may be difficult to obtain in some instances when the patient is confused, upset or unable to communicate easily. In other instances a very clear description may be given, but with a complicated overlap in the story since more than one entity is in fact at play. Finally, the presentation may be atypical and fail to fit the diagnostic preconceptions of the examiner, even after reading this book. The examiner must beware of the temptation to 'put words into the patient's mouth' under these more difficult circumstances.

In general, the patient will volunteer a description of the character of the pain and its location at the outset as the chief complaint. For example, it is quite typical for a patient to answer 'I have an ache in my knee' or 'my sole is on fire' in response to an open-ended question at the outset. To the extent possible, the patient should be encouraged to locate the pain precisely to an anatomic structure of the leg such as a specific muscle or joint. The inquirer must keep in mind the fact that pain often radiates to areas adjacent to its source and that sometimes the source is not in the leg. In addition, pathology in one place may give rise to secondary symptoms elsewhere, as, for example, a sprained ankle on the right resulting in left hip and low back pain due to imbalanced limping. Many conditions, such as arthritis and vascular disease, are multifocal, with variable patterns of prominence among individuals and in the same patient at different times. For example, the location of claudication pain due to iliac artery disease may be limited to the calf muscle on a short walk but also involve the thigh and buttock muscles over longer stretches.

Most often, the character of the pain will approximate one of the descriptive terms listed in Table 3.1. Stabbing pain is commonly used to describe an intense and focal sharp pain 'like a knife' which may ebb to a throbbing pain when less severe. An ache is generally a dull, less localized, and deep sensation. Patients may differentiate between ache and pain, as in 'I don't have any pain, just an ache', at times closely associated with descriptions of stiffness. Cramps may be as intense as stabs, but are associated with a feeling of muscular tightness or rigidity. Shooting pain often comes through as an 'electric shock' down the leg. Burning is a superficial sensation once graphically described when severe as a 'flamethrower'. Dysesthesia, often described as 'pins and needles', usually describes a deeper loss of normal sensation which shades into numbness. Weakness and heaviness are not truly painful, but are common complaints which may surface as part of a pain syndrome.

Temporality is of great diagnostic value but will usually require more elaborate probing by the questioner. The story of the onset of the symptoms fixes the perceived problem in time. The patient may be able to pinpoint an event or moment when the pain began, often with a distinct explanatory cause attributable by the patient. In many instances, on the other hand, the trouble may have started subtly and inexplicably with gradually increasing awareness to the point of sufficient concern to prompt a doctor visit. Circumstances such as trauma, unusual activity, travel, change in medications, and other illnesses are relevant details.

It is useful early in the inquiry to differentiate between constant or nearly constant pain and intermittent pain. Closer questioning will establish the behavior of the symptoms with various activities during the course of the day.

Many symptoms are always present, but at varying intensity depending on factors such as limb use, posture, and dependency as well as time of day, medications, and level of preoccupation by the patient. An important measure of severity is the degree to which the pain interferes with sleep. For example, sciatica and gout are notorious causes of constant misery both by night and by day. Arterial ischemia is also a prominent cause of sleeplessness with relief only by leg dependency which leads persevering patients to sleep sitting up in a chair. Other syndromes respond favorably to some extent to other modifications of posture or activity, with reciprocal modifications which exacerbate the pain. Intermittent pain syndromes usually involve the moving muscular and skeletal parts of the leg and follow a reasonably predictable pattern corresponding to activity. For example, intermittent claudication from arterial disease is brought on by muscular exercise and relieved by cessation of the exercise. Degenerative arthritis is aggravated predictably by weight bearing and mobility, and improved with recumbency and rest. Other forms of intermittent pain follow a more frustrating sporadic spontaneous pattern most typical of various forms of peripheral neuropathy.

Finally, the history must round out a complete picture of concurrent and past illnesses, habits, current medications, and allergies. As importantly, the history reveals a great deal about the patient's reaction to the illness, his own explanation for the symptoms and his likely level of compliance with diagnostic and therapeutic alternatives.

Physical examination

The physical examination should seek to prove or disprove the working diagnostic hypothesis developed during the history (Table 3.2). The extent of the exam includes the lower back, abdomen, and pelvis and may usefully employ the stethoscope, blood pressure cuff, rubber tourniquet, tape measure, hand-held Doppler ultrasound probe, magnifying glass, lancet and culture swab, tuning fork, and reflex hammer. A complete exam will require the patient to perform certain maneuvers while standing, bending over, and sitting and while reclining supine, lateral decubitus, and prone. In general, it is best to establish a routine approach, progressing from standing to sitting to reclining, covering each aspect of the various systems most favorably observed with each posture. Of course some patients will not be willing or able to cooperate fully or may have such compelling preoccupation with severe symptoms and findings that an abbreviated exam is appropriate. Comparison between the two lower extremities is particularly revealing.

Standing

Observation from multiple angles will detect obvious asymmetry in the legs as well as unusual posturing of the patient with upright weight bearing. Side lighting greatly assists in viewing the legs during standing. Twisting and bending at the waist to touch the toes reveals flexibility and uncovers the

Table 3.2 Physical findings in leg pain.

			Vascular		Neuropathic	
	Mechanical	Inflammatory	Arterial	Venous	Root	Nerve
Joint swelling/effusion	X	X				
Soft tissue edema		X		X		
Pulse deficit			X			
Joint crepitus	X					
Joint heat		X				
Joint tenderness	X	X				
Calf tenderness				X		
Reflex loss					X	
Sensory loss					X	X
Sciatic tenderness					X	
Forefoot ulcer			X			X
Ankle ulcer				X		
Cyanosis				X		
Pallor with elevation			X			
Dependent rubor			X			
Muscle atrophy	X		X		X	X
+ Straight leg raising					X	

discomforts of herniated disk, sciatica and arthritis of the lower back and hip. Single leg standing, squatting, Romberg testing, heel-to-toe walking, and pivoting supplement the orthopedic and neurological exam. Repetitive toe-up exercise may produce claudication symptoms and corresponding decrease in ankle systolic pressure and pedal pulses confirming the presence of arterial disease. Venous disease involving the superficial veins is best seen while standing. Inguinal hernia is also best characterized with the patient upright and pain related to the cutaneous nerves of the lower abdomen (meralgia paresthetica) can be evaluated.

Sitting
Sitting with the legs suspended allows a closer view of asymmetries in the calf, ankle, and feet. Dependent rubor is usually obvious, even when bilateral. The ankle and knee joint exams can be completed, along with strength assessment of the thigh and calf muscle groups and knee and ankle reflexes.

Recumbent
Passive straight leg raising, hip flexion, and rotation and hip joint strength are assessed from the supine position. The arterial exam is completed with pulse assessment, ankle pressure measurement in comparison with arm pressure, checking for femoral bruits, femoral and popliteal aneurysm, and distal pathology such as pallor with elevation and tissue threat. Chronic venous and lymphatic disease can be evaluated and comparative circumference at the thigh

Table 3.3 Laboratory assessment of leg pain.

			Vascular		Neuropathic	
	Mechanical	Inflammatory	Arterial	Venous	Root	Nerve
ABNL pressure indices			X			
ABNL venous ultrasound				X		
Elevated uric acid		X				
Elevated ESR		X				
ABNL spine scan					X	
ABNL joint film	X	X				
ABNL neurophysiological					X	X

ABNL, abnormal; ESR, erythrocyte sedimentation rate.

and calf measured. Skin problems can be scrutinized, examining open wounds and ulcers and sampling drainage or skin scrapings. The abdomen should be examined for masses, tenderness, abnormal pulsations or bruits. The muscle groups should be palpated to exclude tenderness, masses or increased tissue turgor. Popliteal and inguinal lymph nodes should be assessed.

Lateral decubitus positions are necessary to assess hip extension and to elicit psoas muscle spasm or inflammation. The prone position may be helpful in examining patients with buttock, popliteal fossa or heel findings.

Laboratory

The initial visit results in a plan for further diagnostic testing as necessary to confirm the first impression or to clarify the relative importance of each component of a syndrome arising from more than one entity (Table 3.3). Some laboratory tests can be performed in the office or adjacent facility at the same visit for the convenience of the patient who, after all, has a hard time moving around. Non-invasive vascular laboratory studies of the arteries and veins, plain X-rays of bones and joints, fluid aspiration, cultures, and blood sampling can usually be done expeditiously with reports returned promptly in many instances. More sophisticated studies such as computed tomography or magnetic resonance imaging scans and angiography require more preparation and may most appropriately be preceded by specialty consultation.

Summary

As a result of the initial encounter the physician should have been able to gather enough information from the history, physical and simple laboratory testing to formulate at least a working diagnosis if not a firm diagnosis. At a minimum, the patient's problems can be categorized by system and by severity to map out an early plan of action based on appropriate priorities.

Table 3.4 Danger signals.

Signs/symptoms	Possible diagnosis
Pain with pallor, pulselessness, paresthesia, paralysis	Acute arterial occlusion
Pain with swelling, cyanosis	Acute iliofemoral vein thrombosis
Painful red, indurated vein with fever	Septic superficial thrombophlebitis
Pain in back radiating to groin	Ruptured aortic or iliac aneurysm
Long bone instability	Fracture
Joint instability	Dislocation, severe ligament tear
Joint swelling, redness and fever	Septic arthritis
Acute paralysis	Cord, root or nerve compression

Depending on circumstances, such plans may entail further diagnostic study, a trial of therapy with return visit, preliminary therapy with referral to a consultant on an urgent or more casual timetable or hospitalization (Table 3.4). The chapters which follow are designed to provide further background for choosing an accurate working diagnosis and an appropriate early management plan.

CHAPTER 4

Mechanical leg pain

Tamara L. Martin, Scott D. Martin

Most episodes of leg pain related to mechanical causes can be divided into chronic overuse injuries and acute traumatic or contact injuries. Overuse injuries usually occur insidiously over time as a result of a repetitive number of relatively small loads. They are characterized by pain, tenderness to palpation, and inflammation. Overuse injuries may produce variable discomfort with daily activities and more severe pain when the activity that produced them, such as running, is attempted. Examples of mechanical pain related to overuse are stress fractures, iliotibial band syndrome, and osteoarthritis.

Traumatic injuries occur as a result of acute massive mechanical overload. Examples include fracture, joint dislocation, and ligament rupture. These injuries are characterized by pain, swelling, ecchymosis, and significant disability. In the majority of cases a thorough history and physical examination will provide the correct diagnosis. Adjuvant testing such as plain radiographs, magnetic resonance imaging (MRI), and computed axial tomography (CT) scanning may be required to verify a diagnosis.

Pathophysiology

Soft tissue injury

Muscle strains represent a tear in the muscle–tendon complex and usually occur at the muscle–tendon junction or occasionally at the muscle–tendon origin from bone. The exact mechanism of injury is still not known but one theory is that the antagonist muscle or muscle group (usually the stronger muscle) undergoes a very forceful contraction while the affected muscle is still in the contraction phase, stretching the contracted muscle to the point of injury. This causes a sudden forced change in the length of the musculotendinous unit, with rupture of the muscle fibers and subsequent bleeding into the tissues. For example, this sequence commonly occurs during sprinting, with flexion of the hip and extension of the knee, which places the muscle under maximal stretch.

Ligaments and other soft tissue components of the joints of the lower extremity are not directly connected to muscle groups and their tendons. They are subject to injury when there are abnormal mechanical stresses placed upon the joint. The stress may be extremely strong, with joint dislocation and severe ligamentous and capsular damage. On the other hand, even minimal stress may produce injury to ligaments and other joint components such as the meniscus of the knee, particularly after previous injury or when the joint is loose.

Fracture

Fractures of the lower extremity are generally associated with severe trauma which may also result in significant soft tissue injury. In patients who are susceptible, such as those with osteoporosis or bone metastases, even minimal trauma may result in fracture. Stress fractures of the pelvis and lower extremity represent fatigue fracture of bone caused by repetitive submaximal stresses over time that exceed the bone's capacity to remodel in response to stress. The most common cause of stress fracture is an increased level of intensity and duration of impact activities such as running.

Degenerative osteoarthritis

Chronic wear and tear with repeated traumatic insult to the articular surfaces of joints may result in hypertrophy of bone underlying the weight-bearing points in the joint, articular spur formation, loss of joint surface cartilage, and a reactive inflammatory process in the joint space. Chronic pain and loss of joint mobility may lead to secondary muscular atrophy and musculotendinous or arthritic conditions related to antalgic gait and skeletal imbalance.

History and physical examination

As emphasized in Chapter 3, the evaluation of pain begins with a detailed history and physical examination. It is imperative to be aware of any history of trauma and the mechanism of injury. In this way any potentially severe injuries that might otherwise be dismissed as trivial at first glance can be identified. Current symptoms including the severity of pain, location, character of the pain (sharp, dull, ache), amount of disability caused by the pain and any prior history of leg pain should be noted. The ability to get to sleep at night and whether the pain awakens the patient are valuable indicators of severity.

Differential diagnostic points must be kept in mind. A history of lower back pain may be associated with complaints of paresthesias and weakness in the leg. In these cases the complaints of sensory loss and pain will usually be in the dermatome corresponding to the level of back pathology. Any history of systemic vascular disease or diabetes should lead to inquiry regarding possible vascular claudication. When pain is related to increased activity, the course of resolution after cessation of activity may provide important clues to etiology. For example, vascular claudication resolves after a few minutes of rest, whereas neurogenic claudication may take a minimum of 30 min to dissipate.

Physical examination should always be carried out systematically, comparing the normal and symptomatic legs with one another. Visual examination is performed comparing symmetry, areas of swelling, discoloration, previous scars, and alignment. The patient is observed standing and walking to detect any evidence of alignment or gait abnormalities. Range of motion, ligament stability, skin integrity, localized maximal point of tenderness and a thorough neurovascular exam including strength and sensory testing are carried out. In cases where it is difficult to isolate tenderness the patient is asked to point one finger to the most painful area of the leg. A thorough examination of the back should be carried out whenever there are complaints of dysesthesias or weakness.

Hip and thigh

Soft tissue
Musculotendinous strains
Among the thigh muscle groups, the hamstrings are the most frequently strained, followed by the adductor and quadriceps groups. Approximately half of the injuries seen in the hamstrings (semitendinosus, semimembranosus, gracilis, and biceps femoris) occur near the proximal muscle tendon origin at the pelvis. Pain and tenderness may initially be diffuse but should be localized within 24 h after injury to the proximal muscle mass. Ecchymosis may be noted at the gluteal fold but is more commonly seen in the popliteal fossa several days after the injury. Ecchymosis distal to the injury is caused by the migration of extravasated blood over time by dependent drainage during standing.

Injury to the adductor muscles is seen more commonly in hurdlers, jumpers and field event athletes than in runners, probably because of the marked rotational forces produced in these events. The adductor longus muscle appears to be the most common injury site. The rectus femoris is the most frequent muscle to be injured among the quadriceps group (vastus lateralis, vastus intermedius, vastus medialis and rectus femoris). Injury to this muscle group is more commonly seen in sprinters and hurdlers.

Early treatment of acute muscle strain consists of ice, compression with an elastic bandage, and elevation for the first 48 h. The patient should also be placed on crutches until ambulation without a limp is possible. Early aggressive stretching should be avoided until the reactive muscle spasm has abated. After 48 h moist heat is used several times a day, followed by gentle passive stretching and proprioceptive neuromuscular facilitation. Eccentric muscle strengthening programs are initiated when most of the muscle soreness has abated. Some studies have suggested correlation of tight hamstrings with hamstring strains and emphasize the importance of fully rehabilitating the athlete before resuming competition.

Quadriceps contusion
Most cases of quadriceps contusion occur from a direct blow to the thigh region. Depending on the amount of compressive force, the injury can vary from mild contusion to severe damage to the quadriceps muscle. When this occurs deposition of bone within the muscle belly (myositis ossificans) can occur which may permanently restrict knee motion and strength. Myositis ossificans usually develops 2–4 weeks after injury but may take months to

show up on radiographs. The ossification may or may not be attached to the underlying bone. The area may be tender and firm to palpation with restriction in knee flexion. Close follow-up is required and malignancy should always be considered in the differential. Maturation of the bone may take up to 18 months, at which point surgical removal might be considered in selected cases.

Symptoms of quadriceps contusion include pain, swelling, weakness, and stiffness which is aggravated by hip or knee flexion. There is usually diffuse tenderness on palpation in the region of the blow to the thigh. Grading of the injury is contingent upon the amount of knee motion and alteration in gait. In Grade I (mild) injuries, knee flexion is >90° and there is no alteration in gait. In Grade II (moderate) injuries, knee flexion is between 45 and 90° with an antalgic gait pattern. Grade III (severe) quadriceps contusions allow knee flexion <45° and the patient has a severe antalgic gait.

Initial treatment is directed at minimizing swelling and muscle spasm. The thigh is wrapped and iced while gentle knee motion within pain tolerance is allowed. Patients with Grade II and Grade III quadriceps contusions are encouraged to weight-bear as tolerated with crutches. Once the initial phase of swelling is controlled, treatment should focus on restoration of motion and a normal gait pattern. Thereafter, patients are started on a strengthening and endurance program. In athletes returning to play a quadriceps pad is recommended for the first several months to prevent repeat injury.

Quadriceps tendon rupture

Quadriceps tendon rupture usually occurs in patients older than 40 years. The mechanism of injury is sudden violent contraction of the quadriceps, such as with a fall. On physical examination there is loss of ability to maintain the knee in full extension with consequent difficulty supporting weight. Usually a soft tissue defect may be palpated just proximal to the patella. On lateral radiograph of the knee a soft tissue suprapatellar mass may be noted with calcifications and patella baja (ratio of patellar tendon to patellar length <1). MRI (Figure 4.1) is usually not necessary except in cases of partial rupture, where a corrugated appearance of the tendon may be noted.

Results of conservative treatment for quadriceps tendon ruptures are poor. Surgical repair should be carried out promptly to obtain the best results. Prior to surgery the knee should be splinted and the limb protected by use of crutches.

Iliotibial band syndrome

The iliotibial band (iliotibial tract) is essentially a continuation of the tendinous portion of the tensor fascia lata and the gluteus maximus muscles. The band passes laterally over the knee joint to insert on the lateral aspect of the tibia at Gerdy's tubercle. It is fixed to the intermuscular septum of the distal femur by Kaplan's fibers. These fibers create a tenodesis effect on the iliotibial tract, producing a taut band over the lateral femoral epicondyle with flexion and extension of the knee. When there is persistent and excessive varus (medial

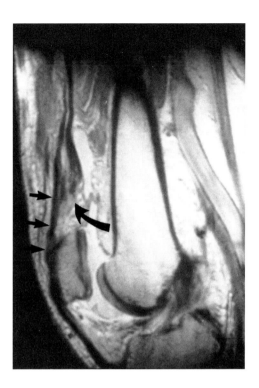

Figure 4.1 Lateral magnetic resonance image of distal thigh and knee demonstrating soft tissue disruption proximal to patella after quadriceps rupture (arrows) and associated patella baja deformity.

deviation of the tibia on the femur) force on the knee, this band becomes even more taut, causing irritation of the surrounding tissues with resultant inflammation.

Iliotibial band syndrome is caused by excessive friction between the iliotibial band and the lateral femoral condyle and is often seen in runners and cyclists. The syndrome has been considered by many to be a bursitis, but it may be a combination of bursitis and tendonitis. It usually responds well to conservative therapy consisting of cessation of the inciting activity for 4–6 weeks or until the area is no longer tender. An iliotibial band and hamstring stretching program should be initiated along with a period of non-steroidal anti-inflammatory medication and steroid iontophoresis with a dexamethasone sodium phosphate solution. Occasionally steroid injection may be required in difficult cases. When prolonged conservative treatment fails to resolve the symptoms, surgery may be required. A triangular piece of iliotibial band that passes over the lateral femoral epicondyle is resected with the underlying bursa. The patient can usually resume sporting activities 4–6 weeks after surgery.

Degenerative joint disease

Degenerative joint disease (DJD) is the most common affliction of the hip among older people, but may become evident in middle aged or even younger

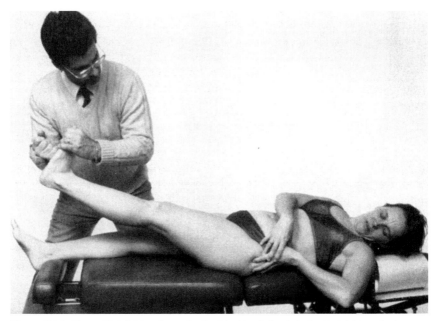

Figure 4.2 Dr Steven Kleinfield performs the Anvil test to elicit pain in the hip joint in patients with degenerative joint disease. Reproduced from Gerard JA, Kleinfield SL. *Orthopaedic Testing: A Rational Approach to Diagnosis*. New York: Churchill Livingstone, 1993, p. 443, with permission from the authors.

individuals who have a predisposition on the basis of previous trauma, infection or gait disturbance which places unusual stress on the joint. Frequently bilateral, chronic mechanical stress results in thinning and erosion of the cartilage covering the bones. Inflammation accompanies this process to a variable extent. Pain results from effacement of the bone surfaces and inflammation.

The history involves boring pain in the hip region with weight bearing and motion of the joint, usually worse at the end of the day. Like rheumatoid arthritis but less prominently, stiffness usually occurs after bed rest or a period of inactivity with improvement after a small amount of exercise. Symptoms are generally predictably recurrent and understandable on a mechanical basis. The pain pattern is typically most prominent in the groin or in the buttock region posterior to the trochanter. Importantly, pain from the hip may present only in the knee region and may be also referred to the back. Related muscle spasm, stiffness or atrophy may produce adjunctive symptoms down the leg and chronic antalgic limp may precipitate contralateral hip, knee or low back symptoms.

Physical findings include pain with various degrees of range of motion of the involved hip joint. The anvil test (Figure 4.2) elicits pain in the hip joint by striking the calcaneous with the supine patient's straight leg elevated. Tenderness may be found directly over the femoral head which is palpated just lateral to the femoral artery beneath the inguinal ligament. In cases with a joint effusion, swelling may be palpable in this region. Motion of the joint may reveal palpable or audible crepitus in severe instances. Plain radiographs reveal effacement and bossing of the femur and acetabulum, with spur formation common at the lips of the acetabulum. Osteoporosis is often noted, particularly among elderly females. Other entities such as slipped femoral epiphysis, avascular necrosis of the femoral head, dislocation or fracture should be evident on plain film.

Early therapy includes anti-inflammatory medications and mild analgesics. Avoidance of activities which are likely to traumatize the joint is helpful, and non-weight-bearing exercise helps maintain joint flexibility and range of motion and reduce secondary spasm. Referral for possible surgical joint replacement is appropriate when symptoms have progressed to the point of unacceptable disability.

Knee

Soft tissue
Patellar tendon rupture

Rupture of the patellar tendon occurs fairly commonly in athletes. Frequently the athlete will have had a history of pre-existing inflammatory symptoms such as 'jumper's knee' and there may be a history of receiving a steroid injection in the area. Often the injury is the result of overloading of the extensor mechanism. The patient may sense a sudden 'pop' while applying stress to the extensor mechanism. Usually the diagnosis can be made on physical examination, with swelling and pain elicited by palpating the inferior pole of the patella. If the tendon is completely ruptured the patient will have difficulty supporting any weight on the limb and will not be able to actively extend the leg against gravity. Usually a defect can be palpated in the infrapatellar region on knee flexion and there may be gross displacement of the patella proximally on the femur. Plain lateral radiographs of the knee show patella alta (ratio of patellar tendon to patellar length > 1) in such complete ruptures. MRI (Figure 4.3) may be indicated in cases of a suspected strain or partial tear.

With complete tears, early surgical repair is indicated. Results of surgical reconstruction for chronic patellar tendon ruptures are not as good as results of early repair.

Prepatellar bursitis ('housemaid's knee') is a common complaint caused by repeated direct trauma to the region of the patellar tendon origin, distinguishable in part by history from partial or complete patellar tendon rupture. It is best treated with anti-inflammatories and protection from recurrent injury.

Patellofemoral pain syndrome

Anterior knee pain is one of the most frequent musculoskeletal complaints requiring evaluation in the office setting. One of the most common causes of anterior knee pain is from the patellofemoral joint. This entity in most

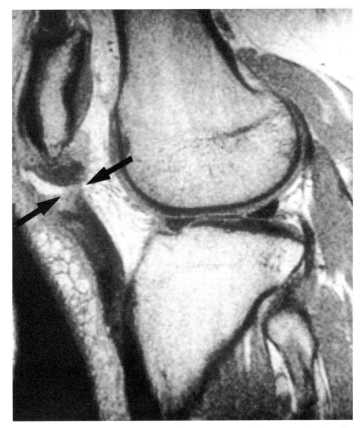

Figure 4.3 Lateral magnetic resonance image of knee demonstrating patellar tendon disruption (arrows) after patellar tendon rupture and associated patella alta deformity.

cases is referred to as patellofemoral pain syndrome or patellofemoral stress syndrome. The syndrome is frequently associated with an increased functional 'Q-angle', or quadriceps angle. Other anatomic factors that can lead to patellofemoral tracking problems with subsequent knee symptoms are a broad pelvis, excessive femoral neck anteversion, genu valgum, hypermobile patella, external tibial torsion, and hyperpronation of the foot. Collectively, these anatomic factors and their sequelae are referred to as 'malicious malalignment syndrome'. A common finding is pain on palpation of the undersurface of the medial facet of the patella. Flexibility measurements are important because a number of these patients have marked tightness of their rectus femoris. This can be evidenced by limitation of passive knee flexion while maintaining the hip in extension with the patient prone (Ely test, Figure 4.4).

Treatment is designed to alleviate patellofemoral symptoms while correct- ing or alleviating any mechanical malalignment if present. For those patients

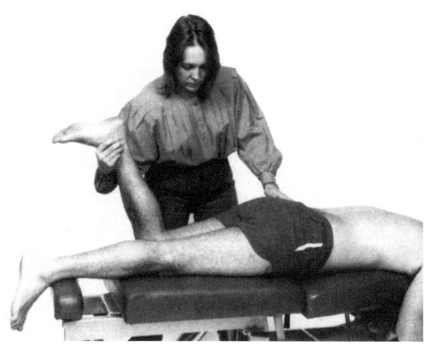

Figure 4.4 Dr Janet Gerard performs the Ely test to demonstrate limitation in passive knee flexion in patients with patellofemoral pain syndrome. Reproduced from Gerard JA, Kleinfield SL. *Orthopaedic Testing: A Rational Approach to Diagnosis*. New York: Churchill Livingstone, 1993, p. 327, with permission from the authors.

with excessive femoral anteversion and/or significant foot pronation, a flexible leather or semirigid orthotic with a one-eighth inch medial heel wedge is prescribed to be worn in everyday shoes and athletic shoes. Physical therapy targets quadriceps and vastus medialis obliquus strengthening, hamstring stretches, McConnell taping for maltracking, and patellar mobilization for tight lateral retinaculum.

Medial collateral ligament injuries
An isolated medial (tibial) collateral ligament (MCL) injury usually occurs when a valgus (from lateral to medial) force is applied to the knee with the foot planted. The injury causes stretching and tearing of the medial collateral ligament fibers and the medial joint space may widen. MCL injuries can also occur as part of a complex ligamentous injury with concomitant involvement of the anterior and/or posterior cruciate ligament, in addition to a possible medial meniscus tear.

On physical examination there is usually swelling and tenderness localized to the medial side of the knee and ecchymosis may be noted. It is often difficult to extend the knee and the patient will prefer to lie with the knee slightly flexed. There is usually some increase in valgus laxity compared with the contralateral side and applying a valgus stress to the knee may be painful. When the diagnosis is in doubt after clinical examination, MRI can be useful. The grade of the MCL tear is determined by the amount of opening of the medial joint space when a valgus stress is applied. In a Grade I tear there is 0–5 mm of laxity, grade II has 5–10 mm of laxity and grade III has > 10 mm of laxity. Testing is performed with the knee at approximately 30° of knee flexion.

Most cases of isolated injuries to the MCL can be managed initially using principles of conservative treatment of soft tissue injury including icing, short-term bracing, and protected weight bearing using crutches. In some cases, however, there may be significant instability and laxity at 30° and mild to moderate laxity with the knee in extension when a valgus stress is applied. This usually indicates complete rupture of the MCL and a tear of the posterior oblique ligament. When moderate laxity is present on full extension, there is usually an associated injury to the anterior cruciate ligament, the posterior cruciate ligament, or both. In these cases surgery may be indicated but will be contingent upon the patient's age, activity level, and amount of instability.

Anterior cruciate ligament injury

Anterior cruciate ligament (ACL) injuries usually occur as a result of activities involving deceleration, jumping, or cutting actions. In jumping activities, the injury usually results from a mislanding that causes the knee to go out. Frequently there is a valgus or outside external rotational force with the foot planted. Sometimes there may be involvement of more than one ligament and/or the meniscus.

Acute ACL injuries are usually associated with a tense hemarthrosis. The swelling may be progressive over a 24-h period. The ACL is partially or completely torn more than 70% of the time when a traumatic hemarthrosis is present. Approximately 40% of the time there is an associated pop at the time of injury. The knee will usually give out, causing the patient to fall.

Lachman's test is very accurate in determining the integrity of the ACL. The test is performed with the patient supine and the examiner on the same side as the affected knee (Figure 4.5). The knee is flexed 20°, and the upper hand is grasped around the outside of the distal thigh while the lower hand is grasped around the inside of the proximal tibial region. The tibia is then translated anteriorly with the lower hand while stabilizing the femur with the upper hand. As with any physical examination of the extremities, the overall laxity is compared with the contralateral knee. False-negative exam may be encountered in the presence of hamstring spasm and/or a displaced bucket handle tear of the meniscus. MRI can be extremely useful in assisting in the diagnosis and in evaluating the menisci, chondral surfaces, and bone for concomitant injury.

There are relatively few studies in the literature comparing the outcome of patients who have ACL reconstruction with those patients treated conservatively. However, most authors would agree that young athletic patients

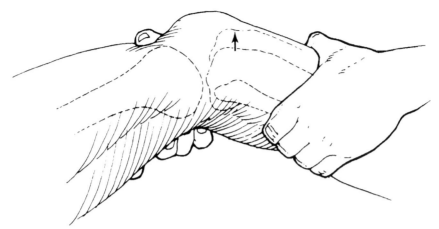

Figure 4.5 Lachman's test for anterior cruciate ligament tear. Reprinted with permission from Feagin JA Jr. *The Cruciate Ligaments.* Churchill Livingstone, 1988.

benefit from ACL reconstruction once pain and swelling have resolved and return of motion has occurred. In these patients the goal of ACL reconstruction is to restore normal joint stability, return the patient to full function, and prevent secondary joint injury and arthrosis. Older patients who are relatively inactive and who have no complaints of knee instability with daily activities may be managed conservatively with hamstring and quadriceps strengthening. In patients managed conservatively bracing may be required for vigorous activity.

Posterior cruciate ligament injury

Posterior cruciate ligament (PCL) injuries probably occur more frequently than realized but are missed on physical examination. The most common mechanism of injury is a blow to the flexed knee, such as commonly occurs from striking the dashboard in motor vehicle accidents or from a fall to the ground with the foot plantarflexed. A second mechanism of injury is a fall with hyperflexion of the knee. Hyperextension of the knee can also produce a PCL tear and is usually associated with an ACL injury and/or dislocated knee.

Isolated injuries of the PCL are often subtle and are thus frequently missed in the acute setting. Usually there is only a mild effusion with little discomfort but increasing pain with the knee flexed past 90°. Physical examination starts with the normal contralateral knee, checking the step-off or distance of the femoral condyles from the anterior aspect of the tibial plateau. The step-off is palpated with the knee flexed 90° and usually measures about 10 mm. Any reduction in tibial plateau step-off compared with the uninjured side is suspicious for a PCL injury. In addition, a posterior drawer test is performed with the knee flexed 80–90° with the foot in neutral rotation (Figure 4.6). Both hands are grasped around the proximal tibia, just below the joint line, and the

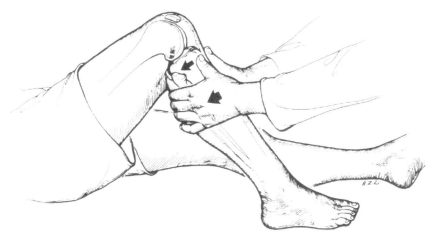

Figure 4.6 Posterior drawer test for posterior cruciate ligament tear. Reprinted from Scott WN. *Ligament and Extensor Mechanism Injuries of the Knee: Diagnosis and Treatment.* Copyright 1991, with permission from Elsevier.

tibia is pushed posteriorly. Increased posterior translation when compared with the contralateral knee is suspicious for a PCL injury. Definitive diagnosis can be made with MRI.

Currently, there is a lack of consensus on treatment of isolated PCL injuries. Some studies have reported satisfactory short and long-term functional results with non-operative treatment. However, most authors would agree on surgical treatment of the PCL in the setting of complex ligamentous injuries.

Posterolateral instability

Posterolateral instability of the knee is usually associated with a complex ligamentous injury involving the posterior and/or anterior cruciate ligaments. If the injury is neglected the resulting functional instability can be quite disabling. Posterolateral injuries of the knee usually result from a blow to the anteromedial aspect of the proximal tibia, with the knee in flexion or more commonly in extension. Often the injury results from a motor vehicle accident or a sporting activity.

Patients usually give a history of pain, tenderness, and variable swelling localized to the posterolateral joint region. There may be a sense of apprehension as the knee approaches extension with giving away into hyperextension during walking and standing. During ambulation, patients with posterolateral instability may ambulate with the knee slightly flexed with a variable amount of internal rotation. There is usually difficulty with cutting, twisting, or pivoting maneuvers as well as with stairs and inclines.

Because posterolateral instability is usually part of a complex ligamentous injury, physical examination should include a complete knee evaluation. In acute cases there may be a contusion with swelling over the proximal tibial region. There may be pain and tenderness with variable swelling over the fibular head and posterolateral corner. The integrity of the lateral collateral ligament and biceps femoris tendon should be noted on palpation.

If gross instability exists with involvement of multiple ligaments, knee dislocation with spontaneous reduction should be suspected. A high index of suspicion of an associated arterial intimal tear should be maintained in such circumstances even in the presence of normal peripheral pulses. Vascular consultation should be obtained with arteriogram in many cases to exclude this possibility. Thorough neurovascular examination should always be performed in all cases of knee injury. Peroneal nerve injury may occur with posterolateral injuries.

In cases of complex ligamentous injury with involvement of the postero-lateral structures, all associated ligamentous instabilities must be addressed and reconstructed if a successful result is to be achieved. Optimal results are achieved when prompt diagnosis and treatment are carried out after an acute injury. Delayed diagnosis or incomplete treatment may result in persistent instability with failure of any subsequent reconstructive attempts.

Knee dislocation

Knee dislocation is a devastating injury that involves complex ligamentous tears and may also include neurovascular compromise of the extremity. The potential for complications is high and may include chronic instability, post-traumatic arthritis, pain and stiffness, all of which can lead to permanent disability. In addition, amputations are necessary approximately 10% of the time after knee dislocation, usually the result of vascular injury.

Description of knee dislocation should include whether the injury is open or closed, condition of the soft tissue and direction of the dislocation. Sometimes the knee may spontaneously reduce, so the direction of dislocation is unknown or the dislocation may be entirely missed. Usually, the knee disloca-tion is classified according to the tibial position with respect to the femur and can be determined on physical examination and by radiographs (Figure 4.7). The most common dislocations are anterior or posterior, with various types of rotatory dislocations less common. In most cases of knee dislocation, both cruciate ligaments and at least one of the collateral ligaments are torn. MRI is valuable in surgical planning by verifying what structures are involved in the injury.

The incidence of vascular injury with knee dislocation is around 30%, but ranges from 16 to 64%. Arterial injury is usually associated with anterior or posterior dislocations but any type of knee dislocation may result in vascular compromise. Anterior dislocations usually occur by knee hyperextension and can result in a traction or stretch injury to the popliteal artery with an intimal tear. In these cases the distal pulses can be intact with danger of delayed arterial occlusion from intraluminal thrombus which forms on the injured intimal surface. Posterior dislocations can result in complete transection of the popliteal artery.

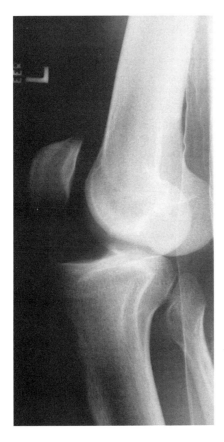

Figure 4.7 Plain lateral radiograph demonstrating anterior knee dislocation.

Management of knee dislocation requires immediate closed reduction with a thorough neurovascular examination. Thereafter, arteriography is recommended in all cases of knee dislocation, with appropriate vascular surgery consultation. If pulses are not restored after reduction of the dislocation immediate surgical exploration and repair should be considered. Observation of a warm but pulseless foot is not recommended in knee dislocation and should not be attributed to arterial spasm. The presence of normal distal pulses does not preclude an arterial injury and should not be a criterion for omitting arteriography. Revascularization of the extremity should be carried out urgently if an arterial injury is present. A delay of more than 6–8 h in restoring perfusion of the extremity in a popliteal artery injury results in an amputation rate of over 80%.

Historically, results of conservative treatment of knee dislocation were acceptable, but with decreased function and an increased incidence of chronic ligamentous laxity. Advances in surgical techniques and rehabilitation have resulted in improved function, supporting increased use of surgical reconstruction in the management of knee dislocations. Timing of the surgery is determined by the condition of the skin, the amount of swelling and whether a concomitant vascular injury exists.

Meniscal injuries

Injury to the meniscus may occur from twisting or squatting or in association with ligamentous injuries from severe trauma to the knee. Medial meniscus tears are more common than lateral meniscus injury because the medial meniscus is semilunar in shape, less mobile and more vulnerable to direct pressure from the medial tibial plateau.

In cases of isolated meniscal tears the symptoms may be insignificant with little pain or swelling. Often there is delayed onset of swelling, which results from synovial reaction to the injury. The patient may complain of recurrent catching of the knee with twisting motions and pain isolated to the medial or lateral joint line on pivoting and/or squatting. McMurray's test is usually positive and is performed by flexing and externally rotating the knee, which produces pain over the posteromedial joint line with occasional palpable click (Figure 4.8). Locking of the knee may occur when the torn meniscus mechanically blocks flexion or extension of the knee. If the separated meniscus is completely displaced in front of the condyle, there may be very little discomfort and normal knee motion.

Arthroscopic treatment of meniscal tears is recommended in cases of patients < 40 years of age or when tears produce symptoms of joint line pain and swelling, regardless of mechanical symptoms of locking or catching.

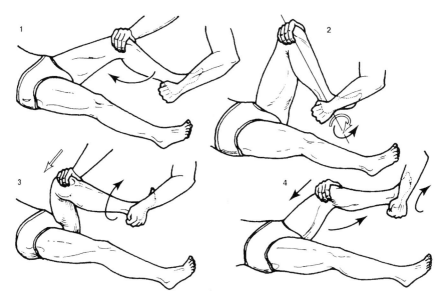

Figure 4.8 McMurray's test for medial meniscus injury. Reprinted with permission from American Academy of Orthopaedic Surgeons. *Athletic Training and Sports Medicine*, 2nd edn, 1991.

In younger patients meniscal repair is carried out whenever possible to salvage the meniscus and hopefully prevent future deterioration of the joint. In older patients, degenerative meniscal tears are frequently asymptomatic and are noted incidentally on MRI done for some other reason. Degenerative tears are commonly associated with chondral defects of the femoral condyle and/or tibia which may produce joint line pain and swelling. When a degenerative tear is present, only the torn portion of the meniscus is removed with trimming of the remaining portion to a stable meniscal rim.

Patellar subluxation or dislocation

Patellar subluxation and dislocation usually occurs as the result of external rotation and extension of the knee with active contraction of the quadriceps. This usually occurs during weight bearing but also may occur in the unloaded knee such as during gymnastics and diving. The patient often hears a tearing or ripping noise during the dislocation. The injury is usually associated with a significant hemarthrosis, with ecchymosis over the medial side of the knee. On palpation there is usually tenderness medially over the intermuscular septum just above the adductor tubercle from tearing of the vastus medialis. Pain is also noted on palpation of the medial facet of the patella which frequently sustains an osteochondral injury during dislocation.

If the patella does not spontaneously relocate, it should be reduced with gentle pressure to the outside of the patella while slowly extending the knee. Compression and ice are applied to the knee and the patient is kept protected, weight bearing with crutches. Radiographs are indicated to rule out a loose osteochondral fragment. Definitive treatment is aimed at re-establishing quadriceps strength while protecting the knee from recurrent subluxations/dislocations. Once swelling has subsided after about a week, active range of motion is started and the patient is placed in a neoprene patellar sleeve with a lateral pad. Quadriceps strengthening exercises including isometrics are initiated early. In patients with recurrent dislocations who have malalignment of the patella, surgery may be indicated if conservative treatment fails.

Degenerative joint disease

Osteoarthritis of the knee joint occurs in the older age group with gradual increase in pain and chronic disability. The pain is focused on the knee but may radiate proximally or distally. Weight bearing enhances the pain and there is usually stiffness of the joint after periods of immobility. Exam may reveal tenderness on joint motion, with effusion in some patients. If a loose body ('joint mouse') from the articular surfaces is present, there may be a history of intermittent pain and joint locking, with crepitus evident on examination. An associated synovial diverticulum (Baker's cyst) may be palpated in the popliteal fossa and must be distinguished from popliteal artery aneurysm. Plain X-ray is helpful in documenting osteophytes, effusion, joint mouse and increased subarticular bone density. MRI is a useful adjunct for soft tissue assessment, including masses in the popliteal space.

Early management relies on analgesics and anti-inflammatories and reduced weight bearing for symptom relief. Physical therapy is important to maintain and enhance range of motion and strengthen the muscle groups which cross the knee joint. When severe or progressive, orthopedic consultation should be sought for advice regarding possible total knee replacement surgery.

Foot and ankle

Soft tissue
Ligament injuries

Ankle stability is conferred by virtue of the bony, muscular and ligamentous anatomy. The lateral and medial malleolus are secured to the talus by the anterior and posterior talofibular (ATFL and PTFL) and calcaneofibular (CFL) ligaments laterally and deltoid ligament complex medially. Varus and valgus stresses are resisted by both bony and ligamentous constraints. Acute injury is often via an inversion mechanism of injury, with or without a dorsiflexion/ plantarflexion component. The patient may report hearing or feeling a pop or snap followed by discomfort with weight bearing. There is usually immediate swelling and ecchymosis. On examination, tenderness is localized over the area of ligamentous disruption along the fibula. Care should be taken to assess the entire foot and ankle, looking for bony tenderness and subluxation of the peroneal tendons. The anterior drawer test is readily performed to assess ankle stability by clasping the calcaneus with one hand and translating the hindfoot forward as the other hand stabilizes the distal tibia. An increase in translation compared with the unaffected side or a significant amount of translation with a soft endpoint may be indicative of ligament disruption.

Severity of the ligament injury is commonly classified as Grade I, II or III based on the extent of the ligament disruption as well as the clinical findings, function and joint stability (Table 4.1). With a Grade I sprain, there is stretching of the ATFL without macroscopic tearing, and mild pain and swelling without functional loss. Grade II sprains are notable for tear of the ATFL with an intact CFL, moderate swelling and pain, and mild joint instability and loss of motion. Grade III sprains are the most severe, with disruption of the entire lateral

Table 4.1 Lateral ankle ligament injury classification.

Grade	Severity	Injury	Clinical findings
I	Mild	Ligament stretch without macroscopic tearing	Mild swelling, minimal functional loss, no mechanical instability
II	Moderate	ATFL tear CFL intact	Moderate swelling, pain, mild joint instability
III	Severe	ATFL tear CFL tear	Severe swelling, pain, instability

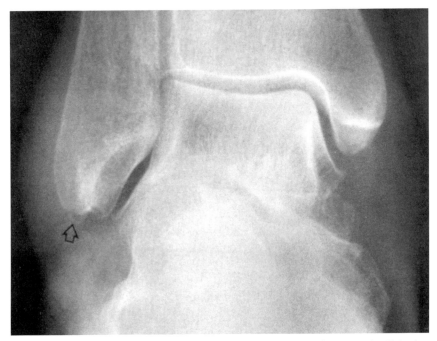

Figure 4.9 Plain anteroposterior radiograph of ankle demonstrating chip fracture at tip of lateral malleolus (arrow) in patient with severe ankle sprain. Reprinted from Rogers LF. *Radiology of Skeletal Trauma*, 2nd edn. Copyright 1992, p. 1328, with permission from Elsevier.

ligament complex, significant swelling and pain, and obvious instability on clinical examination.

Other injuries such as calcaneocuboid ligament tears can mimic lateral ankle sprains. Radiographs may reveal a flake avulsion fracture and clinical examination demonstrates point tenderness over the calcaneocuboid joint.

Radiographs should be obtained if the examination reveals bony tenderness with palpation over the tip of the medial or lateral malleolus (Figure 4.9) or over the base of the fifth metatarsal, or if the patient is unable to tolerate weight bearing. If radiographs are negative for fracture the patient may be treated with an ankle stirrup brace in a supportive shoe and weight bearing as tolerated, using crutches as needed. Ice, elevation and anti-inflammatory agents are emphasized, as is physical therapy to restore motion, strength and, proprioception.

Posterior heel pain

Posterior heel pain is caused by Achilles tendon problems, retrocalcaneal bursitis and preadventitial bursitis. The Achilles tendon inserts along the posterior calcaneal tuberosity. The retrocalcaneal bursa lies just deep to the tendon between the superior calcaneal prominence and the distal tendon.

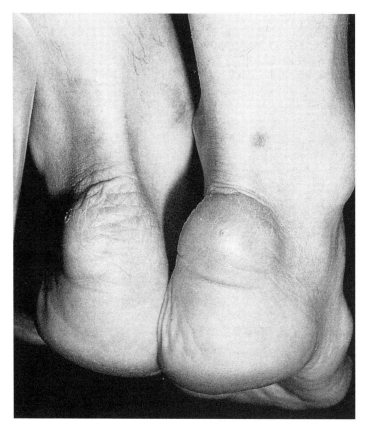

Figure 4.10 Tender prominence over Achilles' tendon ('pump bump', right) associated with pre-adventitial bursitis of the heel.

A less well-defined bursa, the preadventitial bursa, lies superficial to the tendon in the same area, and when inflamed presents as a 'pump bump', or painful prominence (Figure 4.10). Retrocalcaneal and preadventitial bursitis are thought to be aggravated by shoewear friction. Retrocalcaneal bursitis may also be a manifestation of inflammatory joint disease.

Patients present with pain and swelling along the distal insertion of the Achilles tendon, and in the case of preadventitial bursitis a large, thickened fluid-filled bursa is visible. A fluid wave can sometimes be palpated in the retrocalcaneal bursa as well. Shoewear is often painful as the heel counter rubs against the Achilles tendon. Treatment involves rest of the affected area and avoidance of friction over the distal Achilles tendon. In cases of severe inflammation this is readily accomplished with a removable walking boot device or walking cast. Otherwise, use of a backless shoe, low heel wedge, ice, anti-inflammatory agents and physical therapy will usually result in resolution of symptoms.

Achilles tendonitis presents as acute or chronic pain and is quite common in patients involved in running sports. It is usually not associated with an acute injury but represents an overuse or overtraining problem. The patient presents with Achilles pain which may be quite severe, and may be associated with crepitus in the distal portion of the tendon during passive range of motion in the acute phase. Patients with chronic tendinitis may present with thickening and nodularity of the tendon. Treatment consists of avoidance of inciting factors such as impact activities, rest including short-term use of a walking boot or walking cast for severe pain, anti-inflammatory drugs, and physical therapy. Steroid injection is avoided in most cases. If symptoms persist beyond 2 or 3 months, MRI is helpful to determine the presence of a focal degenerative nodule or partial tendon rupture.

Plantar heel pain

Plantar heel pain has been attributed to plantar fasciitis, heel spur, stone bruise and heel pad atrophy, calcaneal stress fracture and peripheral nerve compression. When the etiology is unclear, the term 'heel pain syndrome' is appropriate.

The anatomy of the plantar heel is complex. The fibrous septae of the heel pad taper to an area of looser subcutaneous fat under the arch. Deep to this layer, the fibers of the plantar fascia and intrinsic musculature originate from the anterior border of the calcaneal tuberosity. The first branch of the lateral plantar nerve runs between the deep surface of the flexor digitorum brevis muscle and the calcaneus. Pain in this region may be due to breakdown in the integrity of the heel fat pad, inflammation of the plantar fascial or intrinsic muscular origin, or compression of the nerve. While a plantar calcaneal spur may be present radiographically, its role in patients with plantar heel pain is not clear. No spur is present radiographically in about half of patients with plantar fasciitis.

Many patients with plantar heel pain present with pain on the anteromedial aspect of the heel. They describe a pattern of pain with the first morning steps after arising from bed or from a seated position, and pain by the end of the day after prolonged ambulation. Treatment involves use of a dorsiflexion night splint, stretching of the Achilles and hamstring tendons, and supportive shoewear with physical therapy.

Flexor hallucis longus tendonitis is sometimes confused with plantar fasciitis. Passive dorsiflexion of the great toe at the metatarsal–phalangeal joint reproduces pain in both conditions. Flexion of the great toe against resistance does not produce pain in plantar fasciitis but is painful in flexor tendonitis.

Stress fracture of the calcaneus presents with pain on weight bearing. On examination there is increased pain on medial-lateral compression of the calcaneus. Radionuclide bone scanning of the feet documents increased uptake in the calcaneus consistent with stress fracture.

Compression of the nerve to the abductor digiti minimi presents with burning or numbness along the lateral arch, and may be reproduced with percussion over the medial hindfoot. Diagnosis is supported by electrodiagnostic studies.

Tarsal tunnel syndrome

The posterior tibial nerve may be subject to compression or irritation in the tarsal tunnel formed by the flexor retinaculum behind the medial malleolus at the ankle. The pain is generally localized to the medial side of the hindfoot, but may radiate up into the medial calf and down into the forefoot. Neuropathic numbness in the distribution of the nerve may be the predominant symptom in some cases. In about half of cases, a space-occupying lesion such as a bone spur, ganglion cyst, lipoma or inflammatory tissue is present in the tarsal tunnel. Presence of tenderness and a Tinel's sign over the tarsal tunnel are helpful diagnostic signs. Plain X-ray may reveal a bony abnormality such as an osteophyte in the region. Nerve conduction or electromyographic studies may be useful confirmatory tools.

Early treatment consists of anti-inflammatory medication and joint immobilization using Ace bandage, splint or cast, with surgical decompression reserved for patients with an accompanying lesion in the tarsal tunnel.

Morton's neuroma

Chronic compression of interdigital nerves may result in a neuroma which produces plantar pain between the metatarsal heads. The pain is aggravated by weight bearing and relieved by rest and massage. It may radiate into the toes and has a neuropathic quality. Exam confirms local tenderness, usually in the second or third metatarsal interspace (Figure 4.11). Squeezing the

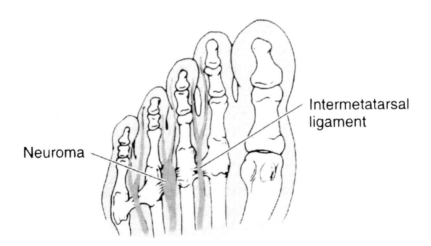

Figure 4.11 Morton's neuroma occurring with impingement of digital nerve under the intermetatarsal ligament. Reprinted with permission from Mann RA, Coughlin MJ. *The Video Textbook of Foot and Ankle Surgery*. Medical Video Productions, St Louis, 1991.

metatarsal bones together laterally may reproduce the pain. X-rays are helpful in excluding other diagnoses such as stress fracture.

Neoplasms

Because of the lack of subcutaneous tissue, neoplasms are more likely to be noticed in the foot than at more proximal locations in the lower extremity. Typically, a mass causes pain brought on by compression during use of the foot or footwear. Bone tumors of all varieties, including rare metastases from soft tissue malignancy, may occur. Osteoid osteomas are most common in the hindfoot, with a classic pattern of resting pain relieved by salicylates. Pathological fracture and swelling may accompany bone tumors.

Soft tissue tumors which produce symptoms include ganglion cysts, fibromas, giant-cell tumors of the tendon sheath, lipomas, sarcomas and hemangiomas. Glomus tumors are most typical in young adults and produce intense pain under the toenail bed. Neurilemmoma involves a peripheral nerve sheath, with neuropathic pain and local tenderness.

Joint disease

Hammer toe

Hammer toe is a flexion deformity which occurs at the proximal interphalangeal joint, resulting in plantarflexion of the middle and distal phalanges (Figure 4.12). When the distal interphalangeal joint is involved rather than the proximal joint, the deformity may be called a mallet toe. Claw toe refers to hammer toe deformity in combination with extension deformity at the

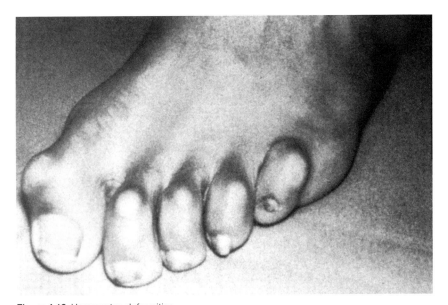

Figure 4.12 Hammer toe deformities.

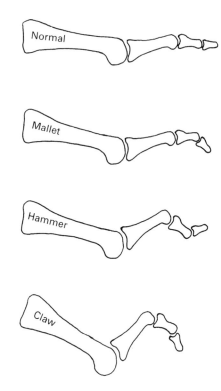

Figure 4.13 Deformities of the metatarsal–phalangeal and interphalangeal joints.

metatarsal–phalangeal joint (Figure 4.13). Symptoms occur on the basis of pressure over the convexity produced by the deformities.

Hallux pain

The most common abnormality associated with pain in the first toe is hallux valgus, lateral deviation of the phalanx of the first toe at the metatarsal–phalangeal joint often associated with medial deviation of the first metatarsal ray (Figure 4.14). Medial prominence of the first metatarsal head (bunion) is the usual focus of the pain, though prominence of the hyperextended second toe crossing over the displaced first toe may also produce pain. Hallux rigidus is a result of arthritis of the first metatarsal–phalangeal joint resulting in pain and decreased mobility of the joint with prominent dorsal and lateral osteophytes.

Bunionette

Bunionette is prominence and swelling over the lateral part of the head of the fifth metatarsal bone. As is the case for bunion, pain is produced by pressure from tight shoes and may be improved by shoes with adequate space for the forefoot and toes.

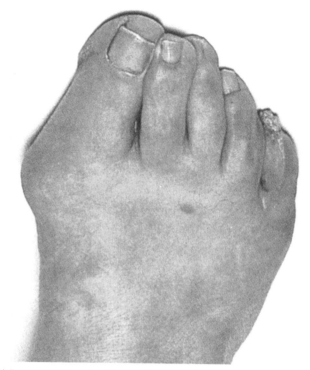

Figure 4.14 Hallux valgus deformity with overriding second toe.

Fractures

Fractures are usually associated with a history of trauma, though stress fractures and fractures of the smaller bones in the foot may occur without a single memorable event. Radiographs of the affected extremity should be obtained, including an anteroposterior and lateral view; oblique views can be extremely helpful in diagnosing non-displaced fractures and tibial plateau fractures. If a stress fracture is suspected, a radionuclide bone scan should be obtained. Although more expensive, MRI is extremely sensitive in diagnosing stress fractures and evaluating the surrounding soft tissues.

On physical examination there will be a variable amount of swelling depending on the mechanism of injury that caused the fracture. Fractures resulting from high-energy injuries may present as open fractures, and special attention to associated soft tissue and neurovascular damage is important. Fractures of the tibia may be associated with a compartment syndrome. As the compartments of the lower extremity fill with blood from the injury, the compartment pressure increases and the leg becomes tense to palpation. A reliable diagnostic sign is pain out of proportion to the clinical findings that persists despite medication. Though verification of compartment syndrome can be made by measuring subfascial pressures, a high clinical index of suspicion and a low threshold for immediate surgical decompression of the compartments is appropriate.

Immediate treatment for most fractures includes rigid stabilization of the fracture site, control of soft tissue swelling, and protected weight bearing. Open fractures and fracture dislocations are emergencies that require prompt attention. Open fractures require surgical debridement and stabilization in an operating room setting. Fracture dislocations must be precisely reduced and most require internal fixation to provide stability. Thorough evaluation of the neurovascular status of the limb is essential. If radiographs document a fracture dislocation of a joint, reduction should be attempted as expeditiously as possible to restore alignment and neurovascular function, then the extremity splinted to maintain the alignment until definitive surgical intervention can be carried out. The neurovascular status should be reassessed following reduction.

Fractures of the foot and ankle should be suspected in any patient with a history of trauma and can usually be identified using the appropriate radiographic views. In the case of calcaneus fractures, plain radiographs may not reveal the extent of the bony injury and CT scan is necessary to determine appropriate management. Principles of treatment include identifying the severity of the bony and soft tissue injury, reducing displaced fractures and maintaining the reduction while healing occurs, relying on non-weight-bearing in a bulky padded splint, elevation of the leg and anti-inflammatory medication. Ideally, surgical reconstruction of a displaced ankle fracture should take place within the first few hours after injury, as delayed reduction of a significant fracture is associated with a higher complication rate. Ankle fractures which are not anatomically reduced and have joint incongruity are more likely to result in post-traumatic arthritis. However, direct trauma to the articular cartilage or secondary chondral wear resulting from ankle instability may also result in chronic degenerative symptoms.

Fractures of the talus, while not common, are noteworthy because of the associated complications. Talar fractures often result from a fall from a height or other high-energy injury such as motor vehicle accident and are commonly associated with other organ or musculoskeletal injuries. CT scans may be useful in identifying the extent of the talus injury and any associated bony injuries. The anatomy of this bone is remarkable for having seven articular surfaces with no muscular attachments. Blood supply is from a network of vessels which form a leash around the body and neck of the talus. Displaced fractures of the talus therefore may disrupt the blood supply, and surgical exposure for reduction and internal fixation may also compromise the vasculature. Reperfusion may follow an avascular incident, but transient osteopenia sometimes leads to subsequent segmental collapse of a portion of the articular surface and is associated with late post-traumatic arthritis. Because of the blood supply issues, urgent surgical reduction of displaced fractures is imperative.

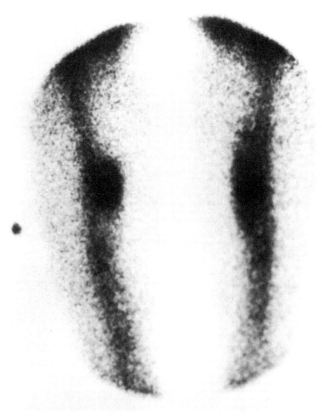

Figure 4.15 Radionuclide bone scan of lower leg demonstrating bilateral tibial stress fractures. Reprinted from Rogers LF. *Radiology of Skeletal Trauma*, 2nd edn. Copyright 1992, p. 1296, with permission from Elsevier.

Stress fractures can occur anywhere in the lower extremity and have also been described in the pelvis. In runners, medial tibial stress syndrome (shin splints), forefoot varus, hyperpronation and tibia vara (bowing of the tibia) have been shown to predispose to stress fractures (Figure 4.15). Symptoms include pain and swelling that increase with weight bearing and impact exercises. Plain radiographs may remain negative for up to 6 weeks due to limited stimulus for endosteal or periosteal new bone formation. In the case of sesamoid stress fractures of the great toe, plain films may reveal bipartite or tripartite sesamoids (Figure 4.16). Bone scans tend to be more sensitive in isolating the involved area. MRI is helpful in evaluating bone for stress fracture and the surrounding tissues.

Treatment is usually conservative with limitation of activities and partial weight bearing. However, stress fractures of the femoral neck have potential

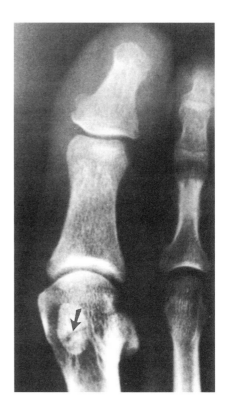

Figure 4.16 Plain anteroposterior radiograph of first toe demonstrating bipartite sesamoid bone resulting from stress fracture (arrow). Reprinted from Rogers LF. *Radiology of Skeletal Trauma*, 2nd edn. Copyright 1992, p. 1511, with permission from Elsevier.

for catastrophic complication and must be carefully evaluated. If hip symptoms do not resolve with bed rest or if repeat radiographs show any progression in the width of the fracture, internal fixation should be considered. Also stress fractures of the anterior cortex of the tibia tend to heal very slowly and may progress, in which case consideration should be given to intramedullary fixation. Occasionally, delayed union or non-union may follow sesamoid stress fractures. Electromagnetic bone stimulators may be helpful in healing such stress fractures or surgery may be required for bone grafting or partial excision of the sesamoid.

Suggested reading

Gerard JA, Kleinfield SL. *Orthopedic Testing: A Rational Approach to Diagnosis*. New York: Churchill Livingstone, 1993.

Hoppenfeld S. *Physical Examination of the Spine and Extremities*. Norwalk: Appleton-Century-Crofts, 1976.

Martin SD, Clancy WG Jr. Knee injuries. In: Andrews JR, Clancy WG, Whiteside JA, eds. *Common Athletic Injuries: On-Field Evaluation and Treatment*. St Louis: Mosby-Year Book, Inc., 1997.

Martin SD, Martin TL, Clancy WG Jr. Knee dislocation. *Curr Opin Orthoped* 1999; **10**:44–65.

Mechelen W, Hlobil H, Kemper HC. Prevention of running injuries by warm-up, cool-down and stretching exercises. *Am J Sports Med* 1993; **21**:711–719.

Myerson MS. *Foot and Ankle Disorders*. Philadelphia: W. B. Saunders, 2000; 1341–1366.

Noyes FR, Cummings JF, Grood ES. Knee symposium: the diagnosis of knee motion limits, subluxations, and ligament injury. *Am J Sports Med* 1991; **19**:163–171.

Renstrom PAFH, Lynch SA. Acute ligament injuries of the ankle. *Foot Ankle Clin* 1999; **4**:697–711.

Rogers LF. *Radiology of Skeletal Trauma*, 2nd edn. New York: Churchill Livingstone, 1992.

Zarins B, Adams M. Medical progress: knee injuries in sports. *New Engl J Med* 1988; **318**:950–961.

CHAPTER 5

Inflammatory leg pain

Sang Cheol Bae, Matthew H. Liang

Pathophysiology

A foreign stimulus causes the body to mount an inflammatory reaction to maintain its integrity. When an organism or foreign protein penetrates the body surface, a series of host responses occurs. The inflammatory exudate containing immunoglobulin, complement components and other plasma proteins quickly appears. Cellular and humoral immunological pathways and the components of inflammation and repair produce widely disparate manifestations developing over hours in crystalline (gout, pseudogout) disease and septic arthritis to years in the case of rheumatoid arthritis (RA). Its clinical manifestations may involve single to many joints to multisystem diseases such as systemic lupus erythematosus (SLE) or vasculitis.

Inflammation varies in intensity and extent and in the particular immunological pathways evoked, but certain features are common to all forms whether it is an acute allergic response or a chronic granulomatous process. Effectors of inflammation exist in precursor forms and are activated. A number of proteins modulate the inflammatory effects and a number of pathways with feedback loops which can amplify the inflammatory process.

Many systemic rheumatic diseases such as RA and SLE are considered to be of autoimmune origin and multifactorial. It is believed that initiating events trigger a pathological process in a genetically susceptible individual in which immune response persists and leads to tissue inflammation and destruction. However, only a fraction of susceptible individuals develop disease. Many rheumatic diseases have strong genetic patterns and others demonstrate polygenic inheritance. For example, ankylosing spondylitis is associated with HLA-B27, RA with HLA-DR4 and DR1, and SLE with null alleles of C4A.

Signs and symptoms

The classic pathological features of inflammation are: pain (dolor), swelling (tumor), heat (calor), redness (rubor). Depending on the tissue and the site involved, some features may be more obvious than others. A joint effusion implies synovitis and points to a structure inside or next to the joint capsule as the cause of the problem. In primary care settings, a small- to moderate-sized effusion in the knee only is likely to be due to microtrauma to the meniscus or ligaments, viral illness, or, less frequently, to early RA or to the spondyloarthropathies.

Some distinctive patterns of synovitis are useful in the differential diagnosis of arthritis. Septic arthritis and crystalline disease of the joints typically affect one joint but can also affect two or more joints simultaneously. The pain comes on abruptly and reaches its maximum over hours to a day. Pain occurs at rest unrelated to joint use and may also be associated with systemic symptoms and low-grade fever. Acute podagra (gout of the first metatarsalphalangeal (MTP) joint) and pseudogout of the knee are classical presentations, but crystalline disease and septic arthritis look identical and infection must always be excluded by aspirating the joint for synovial fluid cultures and examination for crystals and Gram stain.

Synovitis from systemic rheumatic diseases or spondyloarthropathy produces joint stiffness early on. When severe inflammation occurs or is uncontrolled, structural damage occurs and mechanical pain symptoms dominate. Early synovitis causes variable joint symptoms. Patients complain typically of 'good' and 'bad' days. Stiffness is worst after prolonged activity ('gelling'), which improves after using the involved joint. In some patients this can be used to assess the severity of the synovitis. As the synovitis improves the length of gelling also shortens. In other patients with synovitis, gelling may not be prominent or can 'last all day'. A reliable way to ascertain gelling is to ask when the subject awakens and when they are feeling the way they will be for the rest of the day. With advanced disease and joint destruction, pain is constantly produced by anything that loads the joint and relieved by unloading the joint.

Inflammatory diseases

Infectious arthritis
Etiology and pathogenesis
Joint inflammation can result from direct invasion of the joint by bacterial, microbacterial, viral, fungal, and even parasitic infections or as a sterile inflammation in which the organism cannot be isolated or cultured, a group of conditions conceptualized as a hypersensitive or reactive arthritis (acute rheumatic fever, Reiter's disease). Septic arthritis, particularly with acute bacterial pathogens, is a serious cause of morbidity and mortality, joint damage, and functional disability.

Bacteria may seed the joint as a result of direct trauma, surgery, or arthrocentesis, by extension from an adjacent focus of infection, or through the blood from a remote source. Once inside the joint cavity, bacteria can rapidly multiply and cause an inflammatory reaction that is highly destructive to the tissues of the joint space. The most common bacterial pathogens are *Staphylococcus aureus*, Gram-negative bacilli, and mixed aerobic/anaerobic infections. Indolent infections with mycobacteria and fungi cause < 5% of joint infections. Disseminated gonococcal infections with joint involvement or symptoms are common in sexually active patients.

A variety of clinical settings is associated with an increased risk of joint sepsis. These include previous joint damage or inflammation, prior joint surgery, immunocompromised host and bacteremia (pyelonephritis, bacterial endocarditis).

Clinical manifestations and diagnosis

Signs of infection such as leukocytosis, elevated erythrocyte sedimentation rate and fever may not be present, and the only way to make the diagnosis is to culture the joint fluid. Therefore, a joint aspiration is always required whenever there is a possibility of infectious arthritis. The fluid should be cultured in the appropriate medium and a Gram stain should be done on fresh fluid. The yield of cultures or Gram stains depends on the specific infectious agent. In suspected gonococcal arthritis, the synovial fluid should be plated on Thayer–Martin blood agar and put immediately under CO_2 to increase the yield of growth. Gonococcus is recovered in <50% of suspected individuals. Mycobacteria and fungi can be recovered in well over half of the patients by synovial fluid culture, but the diagnostic yield can be increased considerably by doing a synovial biopsy with culture and histology. Blood cultures should always be obtained because many infections of the joint are metastatic infections from other sources.

Differentiating cellulitis from a septic joint may pose a diagnostic problem. Pain from septic arthritis is equally painful in all ranges of motion. Pain from cellulitis hurts most when the joint motion stretches the cellulitic areas. Swelling and erythema in a septic joint occur over the entire circumference of the joint line, whereas cellulitis is more localized. When in doubt, the joint should be aspirated for culture, avoiding the area of inflamed skin.

In a patient with pre-existing polyarthritis, infection of the joint may be difficult to diagnose because it occurs on the background of multiple joint symptoms. When there is one joint that is painful out of proportion to the others one should suspect infection.

Non-gonococcal arthritis is caused by a variety of infectious agents, chiefly *S. aureus*, streptococcal species, and Gram-negative bacilli. Non-gonococcal arthritis generally affects a single joint, most commonly a weight-bearing joint, and especially the knee. X-rays of the joint early on show only soft-tissue swelling. It may take weeks before other X-ray signs of periosteal elevation, bone destruction, and joint-space narrowing are seen. Gallium and bone scanning detect changes earlier than plain radiographs. Nuclear magnetic resonance imaging is more sensitive to anatomic changes.

Gonococcal arthritis should be suspected in any person who is sexually active. A common presentation is a woman who presents around the time of her menses with migratory polyarthralgias and severe tenosynovitis, particularly of the wrist. A characteristic skin rash may occur in two-thirds of patients and tends to be a scantily distributed painless maculopapular, pustular, or vesicular eruption, classically a gun-metal gray lesion on an erythematous base. It requires a careful search to find. Cervical, anal, oral, and blood cultures for gonococcus increase the yield, but some cases are never confirmed and are diagnosed only by their prompt response to antibiotics.

Gonococcal arthritis needs to be differentiated from Reiter's syndrome in men. A typical hemorrhagic skin rash would favor gonococcus. Additional differential points include a preponderance of lower extremity involvement among patients with Reiter's syndrome. Gonococcal arthritis more commonly affects the upper extremity and presents as a migratory arthritis. Achilles tendinitis, plantar faciitis, and uveitis are almost never seen in gonococcal arthritis but occur in Reiter's syndrome. Keratoderma blennorrhagia, a hyperkeratotic skin lesion frequently on the soles of the feet, clinches the diagnosis of Reiter's syndrome. Gonococcal infection of the pharynx or rectum would favor a gonococcal arthritis.

Many viral arthritides have been described, including hepatitis B, parvovirus, rubella, and mumps. In general, viral arthritides result from hypersensitivity or immune complex disease. Clinically they look like RA and have tantalized investigators to link viruses and RA. Most of these arthritis syndromes resolve by 4–6 weeks. Rubella and parvovirus may cause chronic synovitis in a small percentage of patients.

Bacterial endocarditis may be associated with septic arthritis, which is rare, or with sterile, inflammatory synovitis. The latter manifestation is probably due to hypersensitivity or an immune-mediated process. Polyarthritis and polyarthralgias, monoarthritis, myalgias, hypertrophic osteoarthropathy, disc infection, and low back pain are also syndromes seen in association with endocarditis.

Tuberculous arthritis has declined in incidence but still occurs in immunocompromised patients such as AIDS patients, alcoholics and the homeless. Joint and bone infections occur from hematogenous spread and contiguous infection from infected bone. Classically, tuberculous arthritis presents as a chronic insidious monoarthritis with few of the typical findings of inflammation (a 'cold abscess'). The most commonly involved sites are the vertebral column (Pott's disease) and weight-bearing joints. Chronic tenosynovitis may also be caused by mycobacteria species.

Lyme disease has arthritis as a manifestation and is caused by a spirochete, *Borrielia burgdorferi*. It presents with a characteristic skin lesion, *Erythema chronicum migrans* (EM) (Figure 5.1), a red maculopapular rash that expands to an annular ('target') lesion 3 days to 3 weeks after a bite from an *Ixodes dammini* tick carrying the spirochete. EM is often accompanied by chills, fever, malaise, fatigue, and headache or stiff neck. Weeks to months later, neurological, cardiac and joint complications may occur. Joint symptoms occur in about 50% of patients and include migratory polyarthritis without morning stiffness and tendinitis, and they may recur. Chronic monoarticular involvement of a large joint, usually a knee, is uncommon and over time usually resolves.

Neurological abnormalities may occur within a few weeks after EM, last for months, and usually resolve. These include aseptic meningitis or meningoencephalitis, chorea, cerebellar ataxia, cranial neuritis including bilateral Bell's

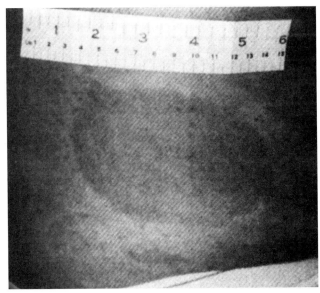

Figure 5.1 Erythema migrans lesion of Lyme disease, 10 days after onset. The outer ring has expanded and central clearing is beginning, creating the so-called 'target lesion'. Reprinted with permission from Koopman WL, ed. *Arthritis and Allied Conditions: A Textbook of Rheumatology.* Philadelphia: Lippincott Williams & Wilkins, 2001, p. 2634.

palsy, motor and sensory neuropathy, radicular neuritis, and mononeuritis multiplex. Cardiac abnormalities also arise within a few weeks after EM and include atrioventricular heart block and myopericarditis.

Management

Identification of the organism is the key to successful treatment with antibiotics. Infections in closed spaces need to be drained. Closed-needle joint aspiration will suffice, except in hips and shoulders, where open drainage is usually required. All suspected or proven joint infections require consultation and hospitalization.

Early on, the joint should be immobilized with splints to help make the patient more comfortable, but exercises should be started as soon as pain subsides to prevent muscle atrophy and contracture. If the effusion does not resolve, joint aspiration should be repeated to reduce the volume of fluid and enhance comfort and full joint extension.

Depending on how quickly the fluid reaccumulates, three arthrocenteses a day to one every 3 days may need to be done. Evidence clearly shows that delay in drainage, particularly delay beyond 72 h from the onset of symptoms, is the largest determinant of whether the patient becomes septicemic and whether there are complications such as osteomyelitis and significant cartilage loss. A joint infection by *S. aureus* can destroy cartilage in 48 h. At the other end of the spectrum, most cases of gonococcal arthritis do not result in joint damage.

A falling joint-fluid cell count and minimal reaccumulation of fluid indicate a good clinical response. Repeated closed arthrocentesis with a needle can produce good results 80% of the time, but one should go to open drainage after 3 days if the patient is not substantially improved and if the volume of arthrocentesis fluid and the cell count in the fluid are not dropping rapidly.

Open drainage should be done early in certain situations. Infections in the hand are dangerous because compartment syndromes may develop rapidly. The shoulder has multiple anatomical compartments and may not be drained completely through a needle. Hips and shoulders always require surgical drainage.

Another question that commonly arises in the treatment of septic arthritis is the duration of antibiotic treatment. As a rule, gonococcal joint infections can be treated for 2 weeks, and all others are treated for a minimum of 4–6 weeks. Intra-articular antibiotics are not used because they create chemical inflammation and because the drug levels obtained by intravenous antibiotics are adequate. Ancillary treatments are useful. Non-steroidal anti-inflammatory drugs (NSAIDs) and joint rest help relieve pain. Continuous passive motion for a septic knee is used to maintain the range of motion.

Patients with gonococcal arthritis should be considered for admission to hospital if there is a frankly purulent effusion, diabetes, poor comprehension and social support or no transportation or home telephone. Effective antibiotic regimens for disseminated gonococcal infection include: ceftriaxone 1 g i.v. daily for 7–10 days or for 2–3 days, followup by cefixime 400 mg oral bid or ciprofloxacin 500 mg oral bid for a total of 7–10 days. Appropriate antibiotics usually reverse the symptoms within 24–48 h. Repeated joint drainage of the effusion is seldom required.

Treatment of tuberculous arthritis requires long-term administration of multiple antibiotics and should always be done with consultation. Fungal arthritis is also rare and has a clinical presentation similar to mycobacterial arthritis. Fungal infections of bone and joint include coccidioidomycosis, sporotrichosis, blastomycosis, and candidiasis. Consultation is suggested.

For the treatment of Lyme disease, oral antibiotics are effective except for neurological and cardiac manifestations. In early localized Lyme disease, doxycycline 100 mg bid and amoxicillin 500 mg qid for 14 days are effective. In patients with allergies to the above medications, cefuroxime 500 mg bid and erythromycin 250 mg qid seem to be good alternatives. Doxycycline should not be given to children or pregnant women. In children under age 12, amoxicillin is effective in divided dosages of 50 mg/kg per day. In cases of penicillin allergy, erythromycin (30 mg/kg per day) can be given. For disseminated infection and arthritis, oral regimens should be given for a month. For neurological and cardiac disease intravenous therapy with ceftriaxone 2 g/day for a month is recommended.

Crystalline disease

Etiology and pathogenesis

Crystal-induced arthropathies is a group of diseases caused by the inflammatory properties of various crystals. The common feature of gout (monosodium urate crystals), pseudogout (calcium pyrophosphate crystals), and hydroxyapatite crystal disease is their clinical presentation as acute monoarticular arthritis. Diagnosis is made by demonstration of crystals in the joint fluid. All respond to non-steroidal anti-inflammatory agents and steroids. Gout responds dramatically and almost specifically to colchicine.

Gout is a disease of middle-aged or older men and postmenopausal women, particularly women on thiazide diuretics. Most patients with gout have onset of the disease after the age of 40. Patients with onset of gout under age 40 may have inherited disorders of metabolism associated with hyperuricemia.

Calcium pyrophosphate deposition occurs in a large number of elderly people without symptoms. About 5% of people of retirement age will have linear deposits in their fibrocartilage on X-ray, and this percentage rises to a quarter of the population in people who are ≥ 90 years. Both inflammatory and degenerative symptoms may occur in calcium pyrophosphate dehydrate (CPPD) crystal deposition disease. Pseudogout is only one of various clinical manifestations in symptomatic patients.

Hydroxyapatite disease has also been identified in some cases of 'acute' osteoarthritis and in persons with acute bursitis of the shoulder and in patients with renal failure.

Diagnosis

The diagnosis of gout should be considered in any patient with monoarticular arthritis, especially involving the first MTP joint (podagra) (Figure 5.2) and other joints of the feet. Polyarthritis is an uncommon presentation of gout. In women, polyarticular gout is almost always associated with thiazide-induced hyperuricemia. Gouty inflammation can be confused with cellulitis because of the marked erythema and swelling, but gouty pain, unlike cellulitis, prevents sleep and occurs at rest. The diagnosis must be made by the demonstration of monosodium urate crystals in the joint fluid.

Hyperuricemia is not gout. Hyperuricemia is a necessary but not sufficient condition for the diagnosis of gout. Although hyperuricemia increases the risk of gout, most individuals with hyperuricemia will never have gout and urate deposition in their tissues. They need not be treated.

Only a drop of joint fluid is necessary for identification of the diagnostic crystals, which appear as needle-shaped 2–10 μm long crystals (Figure 5.3). Large numbers of crystals are generally present in the fluid during an acute attack, and they have also been demonstrated in individuals between gouty flares. The crystals are strongly birefringent and display negative birefringence when viewed with a compensated polarized-light microscope and a first-order red compensator. X-ray of a joint showing sharply defined erosions

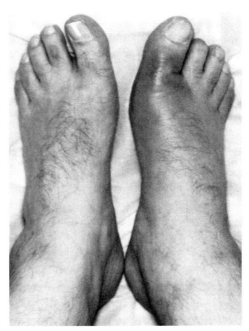

Figure 5.2 Acute gouty arthritis of right first metatarsophalangeal joint with typical swelling and erythema. Reprinted with permission from Koopman WL, ed. *Arthritis and Allied Conditions: A Textbook of Rheumatology*. Philadelphia: Lippincott Williams & Wilkins, 2001, p. 2293.

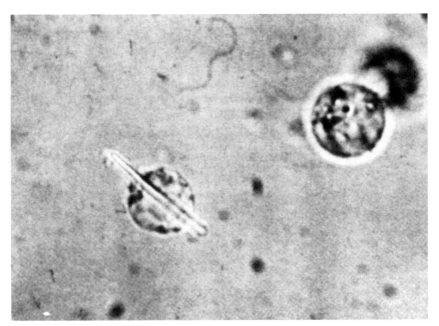

Figure 5.3 Synovial fluid sample from patient with gouty arthritis showing phagocytozed monosodium urate crystal within polymorphonuclear leukocyte. Reprinted with permission from Koopman WL, ed. *Arthritis and Allied Conditions: A Textbook of Rheumatology*. Philadelphia: Lippincott Williams & Wilkins, 2001, p. 2299.

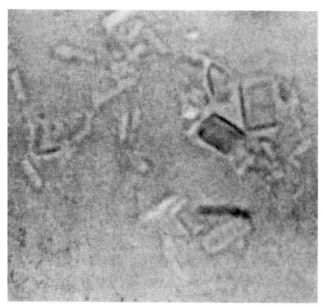

Figure 5.4 Weakly birefringent monoclinic and triclinic calcium pyrophosphate dihydrate (CPPD) microcrystals in synovial fluid sample from knee of patient with chronic pseudogout (polarized light × 1250). Reprinted with permission from Koopman WL, ed. *Arthritis and Allied Conditions: A Textbook of Rheumatology.* Philadelphia: Lippincott Williams & Wilkins, 2001, p. 2348.

of subchondral bone with a bony shelf above is helpful in distinguishing chronic gouty arthritis from other forms of chronic arthritis.

Acute pseudogout is characterized by inflammation in one or more joints lasting for several days or more. These attacks are similar to acute gout, hence the name. However, the knee joints are most commonly affected. The typical feature of punctate and linear calcific densities in the wrist (particularly the triangular cartilage) or the knee cartilage is helpful for diagnosis and the demonstration of CPPD crystals is definitive. The crystals appear as rhomboids or rods, approximately 2–10 μm long with weakly positive birefringence by compensated polarizing light microscope (Figure 5.4). It should be emphasized that infectious arthritis is always a consideration in acute monoarthritis and should always be excluded with blood and joint fluid culture. Occasionally in septic arthritis, gout or pseudogout crystals can be seen as a result of the so-called strip-mining effect.

Management
The severity and course of gout are extremely variable and therefore the treatment needs to be individualized. Some individuals have no more than a few attacks in a lifetime, and others have recurrent attacks with few asymptomatic intervals, erosive disease, and multiple joint involvement, along with deposits of monosodium urate in the soft tissues (tophaceous gout).

Proper management requires that the acute attack be controlled and a long-term strategy be devised. Maintenance of normal uric acid in most patients requires lifelong treatment. It is important that both patient and physician understand the rationale for treatment and commit themselves to monitoring treatment.

The acute gouty episode can be managed with a host of agents, including oral and intravenous colchicine, a variety of NSAIDs, and corticosteroids. Colchicine is an inexpensive and highly effective agent but is also dangerous when used casually. Patients who are older or who have renal and hepatic insufficiency should be given much smaller doses. Colchicine is bound to body tissues and someone who is on oral colchicine must have a much smaller dose of either oral or intravenous colchicine during an acute attack.

For the patient with a fully developed acute attack, 0.6 mg of colchicine can be given every hour until the patient has relief or develops side-effects such as nausea or diarrhea. No more than 7 mg should be given for any single acute attack in a 24-h period, and the total dose should be lowered for individuals with renal and hepatic disease. The best responses to colchicine occur when it is given early. Colchicine may also be administered intravenously, but is not recommended.

NSAIDs (indomethacin, ibuprofen, fenoprofen, naprosyn, tolmetin, sulindac, piroxicam, etc.) are at least as effective as colchicine for the relief of acute gouty arthritis. The maximum recommended dose should be used as early as possible during an acute attack, and when the symptoms have subsided the drug should be gradually tapered.

For persistent attacks, corticosteroids may be required. Oral and injectable corticosteroids are useful adjuncts in patients with renal insufficiency.

Some patients treated with steroids have a flare of the disease after the therapy is stopped, and either a NSAID or colchicine can be used as prophylaxis to cover the withdrawal. The usual prophylactic dose of colchicine is 0.6 mg twice daily, and for a NSAID it is usually half of the standard daily dose. Every drug used in acute or chronic gout—NSAIDs, allopurinol, colchicine—requires careful dose adjustment when employed in the presence of renal disease.

In patients with recurrent attacks and patients with tophaceous deposits with hyperuricemia, there are two ways to lower serum urate concentration: uricosuric therapy, and xanthine oxidase inhibitor therapy to reduce serum uric acid concentration by blocking tubular resorption of urate. To avoid sudden exposure of the kidney to large quantities of uric acid and to prevent precipitation of an acute gout attack, the dose of a uricosuric agent should be gradually increased over 7–10 days in the presence of alkalinized urine. Bicarbonate or Scholl's solution can be used to increase the urine pH.

Probenecid is the most widely used uricosuric agent. A 1-g daily dose results in a mean increase of 50% in the renal excretion of uric acid and a 30% reduction in serum urate concentration. The maximum recommended daily dosage is 3 g. If toxicity occurs with probenecid, sulfinpyrazone can be used as a substitute. Both probenecid and sulfinpyrazone are generally well tolerated.

The most common adverse reactions are gastric intolerance. One should note that administration of salicylates in any dosage neutralizes the uricosuric effect of both these agents.

Allopurinol, a xanthine oxidase inhibitor, in a single dose of 300–800 mg/day, promptly lowers serum uric acid within several days. Doses of allopurinol as low as 100 mg every third day are used for patients with renal failure. It is not a benign drug and can cause liver toxicity, interstitial nephritis, vasculitis, fever, rash, and transient leukopenia. An acute gout attack may be precipitated during the early stages of allopurinol therapy. This may be prevented with concomitant maintenance colchicine or a small dose of a NSAID.

In patients with a history of recurrent renal calculi with hyperuricemia, a 24-h urine uric acid is indicated to determine if they are hyperexcretors of uric acid (i.e. urine uric acid > 1000 mg/24 h). Patients with hyperexcretion are at increased risk of developing uric acid renal calculi and should be treated with allopurinol and not with a uricosuric agent, which may cause acute precipitation of urate stones. The primary indications for allopurinol in patients with hyperuricemia and gout are:

1 Patients who have uric acid kidney stones or excrete > 1000 mg of urate in 24 h.

2 Patients with tophaceous gout who require both uricosuric agents and xanthine oxidase inhibition.

3 Patients who respond poorly to uricosuric therapy or who cannot tolerate the uricosuric drug.

4 Patients with hyperuricemia secondary to myeloproliferative disorders before induction therapy with cytotoxic drugs in whom allopurinol prevents acute gouty nephropathy and renal insufficiency.

The intervals between attacks are called the intercritical stage of gout. Unless the attacks are very frequent, patients with intercritical gout may be simply observed. For individuals with more than two episodes a year, colchicine 0.6 mg twice daily or low dose NSAID can be used to prevent recurrences.

A purine-free diet (essentially avoiding internal organs of animals) may be an adjunct to therapy but is not effective in lowering serum uric acid. Weight reduction may be helpful in reduction of serum urate. Alcohol should be avoided because it both increases production and impairs excretion of uric acid. Medications and clinical states known to produce hyperuricemia should be avoided if possible in patients with gout. These include thiazides, low-dose salicylates, dehydration or fasting, and repetitive trauma.

There are no data that untreated patients with asymptomatic hyperuricemia suffer any long-term consequences other than an increased risk of gout. This risk is small and since acute gout is so easily managed, there is little reason to treat patients with asymptomatic hyperuricemia just for this possibility.

Uncomplicated gouty arthritis is usually easily managed by the primary physician according to the above guidelines. However, in gout with complications such as renal insufficiency or tophi, significant coexistent illness or uncontrolled recurrent attacks, consultation of a rheumatologist is suggested.

Recurrent pseudogout is more difficult. Treatment of associated diseases such as hyperparathyroidism, hemochromatosis, and hypothyroidism may result in diminution of the frequency of attacks. Acute pseudogout can be treated by NSAID and/or aspiration of synovial fluid and intra-articular corticosteroid injection.

Systemic rheumatic diseases (RA, SLE, scleroderma, polymyositis, vasculitis)

A number of systemic rheumatic diseases may have synovitis of the lower extremity joints as part of the syndrome or as a presenting symptom. Practically speaking, the arthritis mimics RA and is characteristically symmetric, involving small joints with a predilection for the wrists and fingers in addition to joints of the lower extremity. RA can present with lower extremity joint involvement alone, but not commonly. For the other systemic rheumatic diseases, exclusive lower extemity involvement would be exceedingly rare.

Rheumatoid arthritis

RA is a chronic systemic inflammatory illness and polyarthritis. It typically affects small joints in a symmetrical and additive pattern. It is an illness that may have systemic and extra-articular manifestations such as rheumatoid nodules, vasculitis, neuropathy, scleritis, lung involvement, lymphadenopathy and pericarditis.

RA affects women two to three times as often as men and increases in prevalence with age up until the seventh decade. One to three percent of the population have RA.

Clinical presentation and course

RA presents in varied ways, and its course ranges from mild illness of brief duration involving only a few joints to a relentless, progressive, destructive polyarthritis with systemic vasculitis. RA may initially present with systemic symptoms such as fatigue, fever, anorexia, and weight loss, and joint symptoms may manifest themselves only later in the course. About 20% of patients have acute polyarthritis and systemic symptoms as their first manifestation of RA. At the outset, no pattern of clinical presentation or laboratory findings is completely reliable in predicting the course. However, poor function, destructive arthritis, and vasculitic complications are more frequent in patients with sustained high titers of rheumatoid factor, rheumatoid nodules, positive antinuclear antibody at any time in the course, uncontrolled synovitis, and hand–foot joint involvement.

Articular involvement in RA is manifested by pain and swelling. Patients with active RA complain of morning joint stiffness that generally lasts > 30 min, but some may have stiffness throughout the day.

Joint involvement in RA is generally symmetrical, although it may not be absolutely so at any given point. The most commonly involved joints are the small joints of the hand, particularly the metacarpal and proximal inter-phalangeal joints, and the wrists, knees, and feet. A small percentage of patients have pauciarticular or monoarticular disease (which usually involves the knees) for months to years. Any diarthrodal joint with synovium can be involved, including the temporomandibular joints, elbows, shoulders, sternoclavicular joints, hips, ankles, subtalar joints, and cervical spine.

Three patterns of disease are recognized: an intermittent course, a long remission course, and a progressively destructive course. The intermittent course is marked by partial to complete remissions and is generally a mild disease. Another group undergoes a long clinical remission after therapy for RA and may have smoldering signs of inflammation, but has little destructive disease. The third group of patients has progressive destruction of multiple joints with disability with or without extra-articular manifestations.

Diagnosis

The diagnosis of RA is made on the basis of the history of swelling, stiffness, gelling, or pain in the small joints of the hand, which is persistent over 6 weeks and may be associated with systemic symptoms such as fatigue, anorexia, and weight loss. The physical examination of actively involved joints shows swelling, warmth, and some pain with range of motion. Early on in the disease, there may be limitation of motion from an increased volume of synovial fluid or pain. Findings such as ulnar deviation, swan neck, bouton-niere deformity, and rheumatoid nodules take months or years to develop. Extra-articular manifestations, such as scleritis or vasculitis, constitute a reason to refer the patient to a rheumatologist, whether they occur early or late in the disease.

The laboratory is not helpful in making the diagnosis of RA, particularly in early disease. The rheumatoid factor may be helpful if it is positive, but the number of false-positive rheumatoid factors increases with age. Between 10% and 20% of patients with clinical RA are consistently rheumatoid factor-negative. The sedimentation rate is non-specific and is helpful only for following therapy when clinical signs are ambiguous. Synovial fluid is inflammatory, but not diagnostic. X-rays are not helpful in early disease but are very useful later to assess structural damage. Six months of active synovitis are usually required before X-ray findings of erosions are manifest.

Therapy

Patient education is of paramount importance. Patients fear loss of function or chronicity and require support. With good care many options exist for control of the disease. Patients can gain mastery of their condition by becoming active participants in their own care, learning how to monitor the disease, use medications, and maintain function by being as active as possible within their capacities. In assessing function, the physician should assist the patient in identifying functional expectations in the context of career, family, and recreation. The patient should be alert to monitoring his overall well-being, since non-specific symptoms such as fatigue, morning stiffness, and appetite reflect disease activity and may herald a flare.

Current pharmacologic treatment guidelines emphasize use of slow-acting antirheumatic drugs (SAARDs) early in the course of disease to have maximal impact on long-term suffering and disability and to ameliorate progressive immunopathological changes which become irreversible. The SAARDs are medications which can heal bony erosions. They include parenteral gold, oral gold, antimalarials, penicillamine, methotrexate, azathioprine, cyclophosphamide, and cyclosporine. Recent novel agents such as etanercept, infliximab, and leflunomide have been approved for the treatment of RA and data suggest that infliximab and methotrexate and etanercept retard structural damage, but their long-term benefits and adverse effect profile are not known. All require close monitoring for toxicity.

Steroids in low doses such as prednisone under 7.5 mg/day and NSAIDs are given for symptomatic relief. There is some preliminary evidence that low-dose steroids may act like SAARDs. NSAIDs do not affect the natural course of the disease. Current NSAIDs have a host of side-effects including NSAID-induced gastropathy. New NSAIDs with highly selective cyclooxygenase-2 (COX-2) inhibition afford protection against gastropathy. Celecoxib and rofecoxib are the two COX-2-specific inhibitors currently available and more are anticipated. Celecoxib has been approved for the treatment of RA, while rofecoxib has not yet been approved.

Referral to a rheumatologist should be made if (i) extra-articular manifestations are present, (ii) the patient is deteriorating, or (iii) gold, penicillamine, methotrexate or other slow-acting antirheumatic drug therapy or steroids are contemplated.

Spondyloarthropathies

The spondyloarthropathies have common features of chronicity, male predominance, predilection for the spine (sacroiliitis and spondylitis) and occasionally peripheral joints, extra-articular manifestations of rash, iritis, uveitis, conduction defects of the heart, aortic insufficiency, and apical fibrosis of the lungs, and association with HLA-B27. These diseases also share a histological appearance of an inflammatory process with predilection for the enthesis or areas where ligaments, tendons, and joint capsules join bone. The disorders include ankylosing spondylitis, Reiter's syndrome, psoriatic arthropathy, enteric arthropathy (with inflammatory bowel disease), and juvenile chronic spondyloarthropathy. The most common are ankylosing spondylitis and Reiter's syndrome. An understanding of these two syndromes and their management can be extrapolated to the less common and related syndromes.

Clinical presentation
The typical patient with ankylosing spondylitis presents with an insidious history of low back pain and stiffness which can be distinguished from garden

variety mechanical low back pain by the history and occasionally by physical examination early in the course. Of patients with ankylosing spondylitis, 20% have involvement of a peripheral joint before their spondylitis. The insidious onset commonly occurs in late adolescence. The most important feature is that symptoms are typically worse after prolonged inactivity (after arising or after prolonged periods of sitting or lying), are improved by physical activity, and are not particularly helped by bed rest. This is different from structural back pain, which is worse with spine use and is relieved by the supine position with the hips and knees flexed. The pattern of hand joint involvement can be useful to differentiate the spondyloarthropathies from other types of inflammatory arthritis. Spondyloarthropathies commonly cause asymmetric diffuse swelling of the digits (so-called sausage digits) or asymmetric joint involvement with distal interphalangeal joint predominance. Dominance of systemic symptoms with fatigue and general stiffness not well localized to the back is an unusual presentation. An occasional patient may present with only iritis and may not develop spondylitis until later.

The typical patient with Reiter's syndrome is a young male with iritis, urethritis, and skin lesions (balanitis or keratoderma blennorrhagia) (Figure 5.5). In addition, patients may have painless oral ulcers or systemic symptoms. Reiter's syndrome may be confused with gonococcal arthritis, and one should consider the diagnosis of Reiter's syndrome in a patient who has persistent

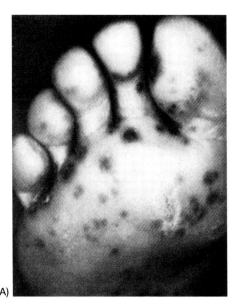 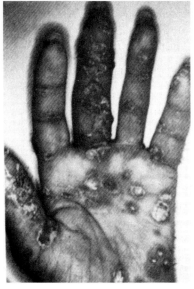

(A)   (B)

Figure 5.5 (A) Early lesions of keratoderma blennorrhagicum on the sole of a patient with Reiter's syndrome. (B) Chronic lesions on the palm and digits in a patient with Reiter's syndrome. Reprinted with permission from Koopman WL, Ed. *Arthritis and Allied Conditions: A Textbook of Rheumatology*. Philadelphia: Lippincott Williams & Wilkins, 2001, p. 1332.

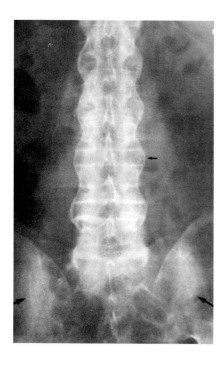

Figure 5.6 Anteroposterior radiograph of the lumbosacral spine and pelvis in a patient with ankylosing spondylitis. Both sacroiliac joints (large arrows) are fused and there are bilateral symmetric syndesmophytes (small arrow) resulting in 'bamboo spine' appearance. Reprinted with permission from Koopman WL, Ed. *Arthritis and Allied Conditions: A Textbook of Rheumatology*. Philadelphia: Lippincott Williams & Wilkins, 2001, p. 1315.

urethritis or arthritis and has been treated for a culture-negative gonococcal infection. Reiter's syndrome that follows dysentery from *Yersinia*, *Shigella*, *Campylobacter*, *Salmonella*, or *Chlamydia* is known as postdysenteric Reiter's syndrome. The typical patient is B27-positive and develops the syndrome within 2 weeks after dysentery.

The natural history of ankylosing spondylitis is good, with most patients being functional, productive, and reasonably comfortable after years of disease. All peripheral joints destined to become involved are usually manifest after 10 years of disease. Patients with early onset or with the hip, knee, shoulder or ankle joints involved are more likely to have worse function later on. The sacroiliitis of ankylosing spondylitis starts in the sacroiliac joints and with time obliterates the joints. It is associated with ascending calcification of the paraspinal ligaments from the lumbar to the cervical spine (bamboo spine) (Figure 5.6). Calcified ligaments can fracture and this is managed as an isolated incident with bed rest and conservative therapy. Spondylitis may also compromise the spinal canal, causing spinal stenosis.

Of patients with ankylosing spondylitis 25% develop iridocyclitis at some point in their course. This is best managed with topical steroids. Patients should be warned about eye involvement and told to report it promptly. Delay in treatment may cause visual loss due to intraocular hypertension, synechiae formation, and occasionally band keratopathy. Patients with spondylitis may also develop pulmonary fibrosis, particularly of the apical segments, aortic insufficiency rarely requiring valve replacement, amyloid, heart conduction defects, meningoencephalitis, and peripheral neuropathy.

The natural history of Reiter's syndrome is generally good, although some patients can have a chronic recurrent course. Their spondylitis, however, does not appear to be progressive. The principal limiting features in chronic Reiter's syndrome are the development of peripheral joint disease and, rarely, disabling iritis or balanitis.

Diagnosis

The diagnosis of spondyloarthropathies requires a high index of suspicion, based principally on the history of inflammatory back pain and with confirmation by X-ray of the sacroiliac joints. It is not important from a management point of view to distinguish between the various spondyloarthropathies early on, since management is similar. The specific diagnosis will eventually declare itself if other organ systems become involved. X-ray confirmation can be done with a simple posteroanterior view of the pelvis which includes the hips. Additional views of the sacroiliac joints may make the diagnosis in some patients with subtle findings, but are generally not needed. Computed tomography or joint scans have been advocated, but there is tremendous overlap between normal individuals and those with sacroiliitis, and we do not recommend them.

The physical examination is not sensitive in the diagnosis of early spondyloarthropathy. The sacroiliac joints are quite deep and are inaccessible to direct examination. Mechanical causes of back pain can produce the same physical findings. Measurement of spine mobility should be done, but unless the results are very abnormal, they are not as helpful for making a diagnosis as they are for following the course of an individual patient.

The two most common tests used are Schober's test and chest expansion. Normal full inspiratory to full expiratory chest expansion should be >5 cm. Limited chest expansion in ankylosing spondylitis comes from involvement of costovertebral joints, which is usually a late finding. Schober's test measures the difference in distance between the line connecting the posterior iliac spine and a point 10 cm above in the erect patient and the distance in maximum forward flexion. However, the test can be abnormal in other causes of back pain that result in paraspinal muscle spasm or in patients with hip disease. A normal Schober is >15 cm.

There are no specific laboratory abnormalities in ankylosing spondylitis or other spondyloarthropathies. The diagnosis of spondyloarthropathy rests mainly on history and X-ray. HLA-B27 testing is marginally useful for diagnosis and does not affect prognosis or management in ankylosing spondylitis. In a patient with post-*Yersinia* Reiter's syndrome, the presence of B27 has prognostic value in that it increases the likelihood of developing syndesmophytes and sacroiliitis. In a few very problematic cases with a moderate rather than a low or high prior probability of having spondylitis, the test might be helpful. Spondyloarthropathies sometimes result in mild elevations of creatinine phosphokinase (CPK) and alkaline phosphatase. In general, the sedimentation rate does not reflect disease activity in spondyloarthropathies as well as in other inflammatory joint disease.

Management

The management of arthritis or spondylitis centers on drug therapy and physical therapy. The spondyloarthropathies are more responsive to the indole-related non-steroidal inflammatory drugs, which include indomethacin, tolectin, and phenylbutazone. Phenylbutazone may be the most effective NSAID for ankylosing spondylitis but can cause agranulocytosis. We prefer indomethacin, which is probably the most widely used NSAID in ankylosing spondylitis. A month-long trial of NSAIDs should be undertaken before its effectiveness is judged. When NSAIDs fail, consultation to a rheumatologist should be obtained.

Microbial antigens persist in the synovium and joint fluid of some patients with reactive arthritis and this has prompted studies of antibiotics. These are inconclusive for the majority of Reiter's patients. A lysine conjugate of tetracycline (lymecycline) hastens recovery in post-*Chlamydia* reactive arthritis but not in post-*Yersinia* or post-*Campylobacter* arthritis.

Physical therapy is a traditional component of managing spondylitis, although its effect has only been studied short-term. The rationale for exercise is to maintain the spine in a position of most optimal function when and if fusion occurs. Exercise that can be incorporated into the patient's lifestyle is most likely to be followed over the long term of the disease. Swimming is an excellent way to extend the spine. Another is to have patients read the newspaper or watch television propped up on their elbows.

Other manifestations of both of these diseases can be treated conservatively. For instance, the conjunctivitis of Reiter's syndrome may be treated with topical steroids. Uveitis, more common in Reiter's syndrome, should be promptly evaluated by an ophthalmologist. Oral ulcers usually require no therapy, but if persistent may be treated with local cortisone preparations. Refractory Achilles tendinitis may require prolonged splinting. X-ray therapy has been used successfully in a few anecdotal cases.

Suggested reading

American College of Rheumatology Ad Hoc Committee on Clinical Guidelines. Guidelines for the management of rheumatoid arthritis. *Arthritis Rheum* 1996; **39**:713–722.

American College of Rheumatology Ad Hoc Committee on Clinical Guidelines. Guidelines for monitoring drug therapy in rheumatoid arthritis. *Arthritis Rheum* 1996; **39**:723–731.

Baker DG, Schumacher HR Jr. Current concepts: acute monoarthritis. *New Engl J Med* 1993; **329**:1013–1020.

Bathon JM, Martin RW, Fleischmann RM *et al.* A comparison of etanercept and methotrexate in patients with early rheumatoid arthritis. *N Engl J Med* 2000; **343**:1586–1593.

Crofford LJ, Lipsky PE, Brooks P *et al.* Basic biology and clinical application of specific cyclooxygenase-2 inhibitors. *Arthritis Rheum* 2000; **43**:4–13.

Emmerson BT. The management of gout. *New Engl J Med* 1996; **334**:445–450.

Koopman WL, ed. *Arthritis and Allied Conditions: A Textbook of Rheumatology.* Philadelphia: Lippincott Williams & Wilkins, 2001.

Luong BT, Chong BS, Lowder DM. Treatment options for rheumatoid arthritis: celecoxib, leflunomide, etanercept, and infliximab. *Ann Pharmacother* 2000; **34**:743–760.

Pinals RS. Current concepts: polyarthritis and fever. *New Engl J Med* 1994; **330**:769–774.

Schumacher HR Jr, Klippel JH, Koopman WJ. *Primer on the Rheumatic Diseases,* 10th edn. Atlanta: Arthritis Foundation, 1993.

Shadick NA. *Lyme Disease, Treatment of the Rheumatic Disease,* companion to Weisman MH, Weinblatt ME, eds. *Textbook of Rheumatology.* Philadelphia: W.B. Saunders Co., 1995.

CHAPTER 6

Vascular leg pain

Magruder C. Donaldson

Pathophysiology

Lower extremity pain can arise from abnormalities in either arteries or veins. In the case of arterial disease, the tissues are insufficiently supplied with oxygenated blood because of obstruction to inflow. In the case of veins, valvular incompetence or venous obstruction result in distention and excessive hydrostatic pressure in the veins and adjacent tissues. In rare instances, virtually total venous obstruction may result in sufficient reduction in outflow of blood to seriously reduce nutrient capillary inflow, resulting in tissue ischemia.

Arterial flow is capable of increasing dramatically in response to demand. During muscle contraction as with walking, metabolic byproducts build up in the muscles resulting in reflex vasodilatation and reduced vascular resistance. Compensatory inflow rapidly follows to nourish the exercising muscle. In the presence of arterial obstructive disease, compensatory inflow is retarded and the increased demands cannot be met. Ischemic claudication pain ensues which persists until demand is reduced by cessation of exercise and the supply of oxygenated blood can be replenished.

Obstruction of the main arterial channels results in enlargement of collaterals connecting the proximal relatively undiseased arterial tree with the distal underperfused tree. If the occlusion is limited to a relatively short segment of artery, such as the iliac or superficial femoral, collateral channels can usually provide sufficient flow into the distal tree to render the leg symptom-free until exercise increases demand. Such segmental disease causing intermittent claudication generally reduces the resting systolic pressure ratio between the ankle and the arm to 0.4–0.9. In situations where there are multiple obstructions in series, such as combined iliac and femoral disease, collateral flow must bridge a longer distance, with reduced blood pressure and flow to the distal bed. Such patterns, as well as patterns of severe obstruction in the more distal portion of the leg below the knee, account for most instances of ischemic pain at rest. Resting ischemic symptoms and findings are generally associated with ankle/brachial pressure ratios <0.4. With acute occlusion of an essentially normal artery, there are no enlarged collaterals available at the onset of ischemia and the severity of ischemia is consequently greater than in more chronic situations where obstruction develops slowly and collaterals have had sufficient time to enlarge. Ischemia results in pain, progressing to paresthesia and numbness and finally to paralysis due to both nerve and muscle involvement as the duration and severity of ischemia increase. Symptoms of chronic arterial occlusive disease may be enhanced in the presence of anemia and reduced cardiac output.

Acute venous occlusion results in abrupt increase in pressure in veins distal to the obstruction. Collaterals naturally enlarge to carry flow into the lower pressure venous tree proximal to the obstruction. Increased pressure produces distension of the veins and increases interstitial fluid within the muscle compartments causing painful stretching of the fascia. In the presence of acute thrombosis, variable associated inflammation of the vein adjacent to thrombus adds a component of inflammatory pain. When venous outflow is virtually completely obstructed through both main channels and adjacent collaterals, as in *Phlegmasia alba dolens*, arterial inflow is impeded sufficiently to produce ischemic pain. With more chronic obstruction, pain is generally minimal because of the absence of inflammation and presence of large collaterals which decompress the distal veins. In some circumstances, however, sufficient venous obstruction may be present to produce intermittent claudication based on inability of the venous tract to provide sufficient outflow for the increased amounts of arterial inflow brought on by muscle contraction. Most commonly, chronic venous insufficiency on the basis of primary valvular incompetence or previous deep vein thrombosis (DVT) results in enlargement of venous channels, increased hydrostatic pressure in the more distal portion of the leg with dependence and pressure transmission to the fascia and superficial tissues with consequent sensations of heaviness, stretching, and aching.

Arterial disease

Acute arterial occlusion
Presentation
Acute arterial occlusion results in sudden, abrupt onset of peripheral ischemic pain. The level of severity is generally extreme, but may be relatively mild in cases of arterial thrombosis superimposed upon chronic peripheral vascular disease (PVD). The most common etiology of acute obstruction (Table 6.1) is an embolus from the heart which lodges at a major bifurcation in the arterial tree, simultaneously obstructing both the main channel and the most important collateral for that channel. Another dramatic etiology is abrupt thrombosis of a popliteal aneurysm, during which a chronic laminar thrombus lining the aneurysm wall becomes disrupted with peripheral embolization or obstruction at the site of the aneurysm. More rarely, abdominal aortic, iliac or femoral aneurysm may produce acute obstruction by a similar mechanism. In the presence of chronic PVD, underlying arterial stenoses may abruptly progress to total thrombotic occlusion. A notable change in the pattern of chronic ischemic symptoms results, but usually in a less dramatic fashion than in patients with little PVD because of the presence of preconditioned collateral channels.

Table 6.1 Causes of acute lower extremity arterial occlusion.

Arterial thromboembolism
Valvular heart disease with vegetation/thrombus on leaflet
Left ventricular aneurysm with thrombus
Atrial fibrillation/left atrial enlargement with thrombus
Left ventricular mural thrombus following myocardial infarction
Paradoxical embolus through patent foramen ovale
Tumor embolus (atrial myxoma, tumor in pulmonary vein)
Aortic aneurysm thrombus disruption
Peripheral (femoral, popliteal) aneurysm

Arterial thrombosis
Hypercoagulable states
Severe systemic illness (sepsis, cardiovascular collapse, trauma)
Iatrogenic arterial injury (catheters, wires)
Trauma
Plaque rupture
Peripheral bypass thrombosis

Table 6.2 Differential diagnosis of arterial embolus vs. thrombosis.

	Embolus	Thrombus
Identifiable source	Usually cardiac disease	Less common
Severity of ischemia	Usually profound	Commonly less severe
Course over hours	Usual improvement	Little improvement
History of leg PVD	Less common	Common
Chronic PVD signs	Few; other leg normal	Common; other leg abnormal
Arteriography	Scant disease, few collaterals	Diffuse disease, many collaterals

PVD, Peripheral vascular disease.

Diagnostic differentiation between embolus and thrombosis is important, though sometimes difficult (Table 6.2). Historical features of embolus include dramatic onset without antecedent chronic peripheral arterial symptoms and the presence of cardiac valvular disease, recent myocardial infarction or arrhythmia. In addition, patients with acute embolic occlusion will often experience some improvement over the first few hours after onset as new collaterals are solicited. Acute thrombosis with underlying PVD is associated with a history of chronic arterial symptoms such as claudication. There may be less improvement over the first hours after an abrupt event because collateral has already developed near maximally. Aneurysms are generally asymptomatic without any useful historical clues, though the patient may have been aware of an unusual pulsation in retrospect.

The level of tissue ischemia is reflected in the signs and symptoms (Table 6.3). If the symptoms are unilateral, comparison with the more normal contralateral leg is helpful. Pain is the cardinal early symptom of ischemia.

Table 6.3 Signs and symptoms of acute arterial occlusion.

Pain
Pulselessness
Pallor
Paresthesia
Paralysis

With prolongation, numbness and paresthesia supervene followed by loss of motor function. Physical examination will reveal pallor in the ischemic portion of the limb. Capillary and venous filling times will be prolonged and marked blanching will occur with elevation. A sensory deficit may be present, corresponding to the patient's symptoms. The distal limb may improve with time as collateral channels are recruited, with most dramatic restoration of capillary filling and warmth in cases of acute occlusion in the absence of underlying PVD. Pulses will be absent below the level of obstruction. Paradoxically, the pulses above the level of obstruction may be abnormally prominent as flow is frustrated at the point of occlusion, a variant of the so-called 'water hammer pulse'. There may be evidence of abdominal, iliac, femoral or popliteal aneurysm on palpation. Arrhythmia may be evident or there may be other signs of cardiac disease such as peripheral edema, gallops, cardiac enlargement or rales.

Laboratory
The hand-held Doppler probe is an excellent adjunct to extend the usefulness of the physical examination. It can be used in the office to obtain systolic blood pressure at the ankle (Figure 6.1), which when compared with the brachial pressure yields the ankle–brachial index. More formal non-invasive vascular laboratory confirmation with segmental limb pressures and pulse volume recordings provides a relatively precise measure of the presence and degree of arterial disease (Figure 6.2), but is generally not necessary to the initial diagnosis, particularly in acute situations when the history and physical usually tell the story so clearly. Ultrasound imaging, computed tomography or magnetic resonance imaging (MRI) can prove the presence of an abdominal or peripheral aneurysm. Arteriography can identify the exact level of obstruction and help plan definitive therapy. Electrocardiogram and echocardiography help elucidate underlying contributory cardiac disease.

Management
The most important step in early management of patients with acute arterial occlusion is making a timely diagnosis. In the absence of contraindications, anticoagulation with intravenous heparin is an appropriate early step to protect collateral from propagation of secondary thrombosis around the acute obstruction and to help protect the patient from repeat embolic episodes. The patient should be postured in the foot down, reverse Trendelenberg position

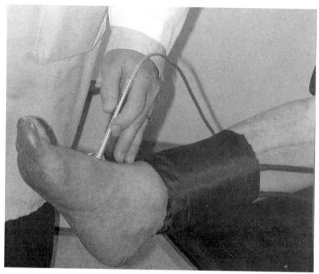

Figure 6.1 Office use of hand-held Doppler probe to detect pedal artery flow to obtain systolic blood pressure at the ankle. Once flow is detected, the cuff is inflated until flow stops. The cuff is then slowly deflated and pressure read at the point when flow is first detected by the probe. Prompt comparison with brachial blood pressure allows calculation of the ankle–brachial pressure index ratio for later reference.

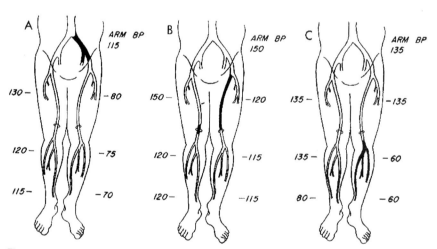

Figure 6.2 Patterns of segmental limb pressures with various combinations of peripheral arterial occlusive disease. (A) Left iliac artery occlusion with uniformly depressed pressures in thigh, calf and ankle locations compared with the right side and arm. (B) Bilateral superficial femoral disease, with short distal occlusion in the right leg and diffuse occlusion on the left producing associated pressure deficits. (C) Bilateral occlusions below the knee joint, with distal disease in the right leg and more diffuse disease on the left with associated patterns of pressure deficits.

to take advantage of gravity to augment flow into the distal arterial bed. The heels and forefeet should be protected from mechanical trauma. The fascial compartments should be monitored for development of compartment syndrome with secondary injury to nerve and muscle produced by increased subfascial pressure. Underlying cardiac disease should be aggressively managed with appropriate consultation, particularly if a new event such as myocardial infarction or arrhythmia is evolving simultaneously. In virtually all cases, early consultation to general or vascular surgery should be sought. If the limb is restored to a fully sensate and pain-free status, no definitive early therapy may be required. With persistent pain, and most particularly with progressive or persistent numbness, urgent intervention is paramount, using either percutaneous thrombectomy/fibrinolysis, surgery or a combination of the two modalities to establish improved flow.

Chronic arterial occlusion
Presentation
Though chronic atherosclerotic peripheral occlusive disease can present in patients < 50 years of age, it generally appears later in life and follows a relatively gradual pattern of progression as thickening of the arterial wall eventually produces occlusion. Whether localized to the aortoiliac, superficial femoral or infrapopliteal arteries or to a combination of these three segments, disease is most often initially manifest by onset of intermittent claudication. The critical historical feature of intermittent claudication is repetitive stereotypical pain brought on after initiation of exercise with relief upon cessation of exercise. Muscle cramping and fatigue develop after a generally reproducible amount of exercise with prompt relief after stopping to stand or sit. With prolongation of exercise, the symptoms may evolve into numbness or even paralysis and relief may be delayed with some residual aching and even tenderness in the muscle. As in angina pectoris, symptoms are aggravated by added demand such as walking rapidly, walking up an incline or carrying heavy bundles.

The most common situation involves unilateral stenosis or occlusion of the superficial femoral artery producing calf muscle pain. The pattern of claudication may extend to the thigh and buttock musculature if the aorta or iliac arteries are diseased, though relatively isolated calf symptoms may predominate if exercise is not prolonged. Male patients with aortoiliac disease may complain of impotence in addition to bilateral buttock, thigh, and calf claudication (the 'LeRiche syndrome'). In unusual patients with severe involvement of the internal iliac arteries and relative sparing of the main iliac and femoral trunks, impotence may be present with claudication limited to the buttock muscles. A predominance of disease in the tibial segment of the leg can produce claudication limited to the ankle and foot.

With progression to a more severe level, PVD results in ischemic symptoms at rest. Resting symptoms usually imply involvement of either multiple proximal arterial segments, such as combined iliac and femoral disease, or a predominance of isolated distal disease in the tibial vessels. Historically, the first manifestation of resting ischemia is often nocturnal. With recumbency and sleep, heart rate and blood pressure are reduced and flow into the most peripheral portions of the diseased arterial tree is diminished. Typically, a few hours after bedtime the patient will be awakened by numbness, tingling or aching pain in the toes and forefoot. This discomfort is relieved by dependency, produced by sitting at the edge of the bed or by standing or walking around for a short time. Many patients learn that they can sleep most comfortably sitting in a chair or with the bed tipped in a foot down position.

It is a short distance between nocturnal symptomatology and a more constant pattern of resting ischemia. Typically, the pain is a combination of aching and a neuropathic syndrome involving paresthesias and numbness. The pain is generally relieved to some extent by leg dependency and aggravated by elevation. Walking and standing will be uncomfortable because of pressure on the ischemic extremity and superimposition of muscular ischemia during muscle contraction. A slight injury, crack or other inadvertent trauma will easily produce an open non-healing lesion with attendant inflammation and potential for secondary infection. These lesions predominate in the most distal portion of the foot and on the areas such as toe tips, bony prominences, and nails subject to contact and injury.

Physical examination reveals reduced or absent peripheral pulses. In rare instances, a patient with mild claudication based on arterial stenosis may have a normal pulse exam at rest. After a period of exercise such as walking or repetitive tiptoe ankle flexion while standing sufficient to bring on claudication, prompt re-examination should reveal reduction or absence of pulses in the involved extremity. With strictly unilateral symptoms it is valuable to compare findings with the uninvolved extremity, realizing that the asymptomatic limb may not be entirely normal but simply masked by the more diseased limb. More severe levels of chronic disease produce muscle atrophy on the basis of poor nutrition and lack of use. Similarly, the skin over the foot is cool, shiny, dry, and atrophic with advanced chronic disease. The absence of hair over the ankle and toes is non-specific and never an isolated finding. Profound pallor with elevation (Figure 6.3) with delayed filling of the forefoot veins beyond 20 s on return of the leg to the horizontal position should accompany resting symptoms. Capillary filling time is delayed when elicited by pressing the skin to empty the capillaries and observing the promptness with which the blanching disappears after release of pressure. With leg dependency, rubor over the distal portion of the foot may be striking, indicating loss of vasomotor tone in the subdermal plexus in the face of advanced ischemia (Figure 6.4). Cyanosis may also occur if there is coincident venous disease or extremely sluggish flow. Open lesions or non-healing minor injuries are distributed generally in the most distal portion of the foot or at contact areas such as the heel or metatarsal heads. Peripheral edema may be present in patients in whom peripheral ischemia is sufficiently severe to require dependency for relief. Such edema may be enhanced when skin breakdown has produced inflammation and infection.

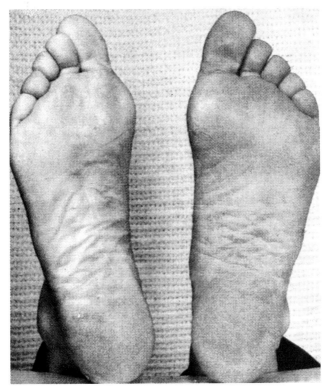

Figure 6.3 Pallor of patient's right foot with elevation in comparison with normal left foot. Adapted from Walker WF. *Color Atlas of Peripheral Vascular Diseases*. Copyright 1980, p. 26, with permission from Elsevier.

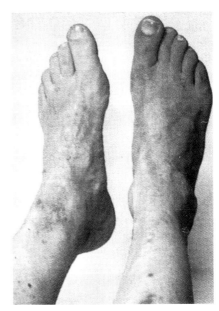

Figure 6.4 Rubor of patient's right foot with dependency in comparison with normal left foot. Adapted from Walker WF. *Color Atlas of Peripheral Vascular Diseases*. Copyright 1980, p. 26, with permission from Elsevier.

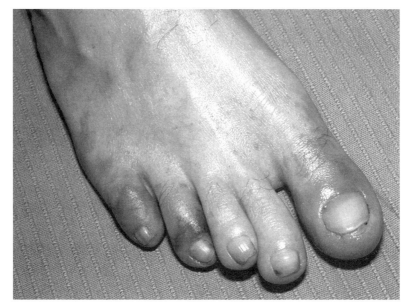

Figure 6.5 'Blue toe syndrome' resulting from atheroembolism to the foot from a proximal atherosclerotic plaque. Note distal distribution in variegated pattern corresponding to digital artery branch occlusions.

Variants and differential points

Acute manifestations may be superimposed upon a history of chronic disease. For example, abrupt embolization of atheromatous material or small bits of thrombus from a stenotic region of the aorta, iliac or femoral artery can produce the so-called 'blue toe syndrome'. The typical history involves no antecedent arterial symptoms or mild claudication consistent with proximal stenosis, with abrupt onset of painful mottled discoloration over the distal portion of the ipsilateral foot or one or more toes (Figure 6.5) consistent with abrupt embolic occlusion of a digital artery or the plantar artery by atheromatous debris which has dislodged from a proximal plaque.

Other varieties of chronic arterial disease include Buerger's disease (*Thromboangiitis obliterans*) in which pruning of the pedal and tibial vessels occurs. The classic presentation is a young male smoker with ischemic lesions distributed distally, typically with palpable pulses to the level of the popliteal artery but none more distally. A similar distal distribution is common in another variant of PVD seen in patients with diabetes in whom isolated calcific arterial occlusive disease is present in the tibial arteries, usually with relative sparing of the pedal vessels. Many diabetics also have more proximal arterial disease. Peripheral neuropathy is a prominent feature among diabetic patients with or without accompanying arterial occlusive disease, producing *mal perforans* ulcers over areas of weight bearing such as the metatarsal heads.

Diabetics frequently present with purely neuropathic ulceration with bounding pedal pulses. Vasospastic conditions present with a history of cold sensitivity and there may be objective evidence of accompanying systemic collagen vascular disease. It is very uncommon to have tissue loss in the presence of vasospasm alone without arterial occlusion. Vasculitis may result in digital artery occlusion, producing ischemic lesions and digital gangrene. Patients who present at < 50 years are particularly challenging, since the differential diagnosis includes adventitial cystic disease of the popliteal artery, popliteal artery entrapment syndrome and exercise-induced compartment syndrome. In addition, such young patients often harbor a particularly virulent brand of arterial disease which may be associated with hypercoagulable states and multiple risk factors for systemic atherosclerosis.

True intermittent claudication is predominantly of arterial origin. Symptoms very similar to aortoiliac arterial claudication may be produced by spinal stenosis, with a proximal distribution of pain and other historical and physical findings which must be carefully sorted through to make an accurate differential diagnosis (see Chapter 7). Spinal stenosis generally produces more of a diffuse numbing weakness than a muscular cramping fatigue. Distress may be caused by simple standing or other postures which increase lumbar lordosis and may persist long after walking ceases with best relief by sitting or other maneuvers which allow lumbar spine flexion. Other neuropathic symptoms are often present, such as perineal numbness or tingling. Venous obstruction is also an unusual cause of intermittent claudication (see below).

Laboratory

Confirmatory laboratory consists largely of physiological non-invasive vascular studies. At rest, the presence of significant peripheral arterial occlusive disease almost always causes abnormalities in segmental limb pressure and pulse volume recordings. Non-compliant or calcified arteries may be non-compressible, resulting in unmeasurable or falsely elevated segmental limb pressures. The minority of patients complaining of claudication but with normal physical and laboratory findings at rest may need treadmill exercise study to elicit symptoms and associated changes in segmental limb pressures to clarify the diagnosis and differentiate arterial disease from other etiologies such as spinal stenosis. Anatomic imaging with MRI or contrast angiography are rarely necessary to make the diagnosis of PVD and should be reserved until after consultation with vascular specialists for patients with severe disease who may be candidates for intervention.

Management

Early management strategy depends on presentation. In the case of intermittent claudication, the patient should be advised to initiate a daily exercise regimen. Walking to the point of discomfort, with cessation until comfort returns followed by repeat cycles, usually produces improved collateral flow as well as metabolic adaptation of the muscle itself. Symptoms stabilize or improve in as many as 80% of patients. The addition of pentoxyphyllin or cilostazol has been proven to enhance the likelihood of improvement in most studies, though the degree of improvement for any given individual is unpredictable. A trial of pharmacotherapy may be worthwhile in cases where the risk of intervention is substantial or in individuals in whom the ability to walk an additional short distance would make an important difference to lifestyle. Patients should be cautioned about proper foot care and vigorous efforts should be made to address underlying risk factors such as homocysteinemia, hyperlipidemia, hypertension, diabetes, smoking, and obesity. If the history and physical examination suggest the presence of stenosis in the iliac or superficial femoral artery, percutaneous therapy with balloon angioplasty or stent may be a relatively simple and reasonable therapeutic option. In such selected circumstances, early referral for scan or arteriography is appropriate. In most circumstances, referral for intervention is not warranted unless the claudication is truly disabling or progresses to resting ischemia. Only 3–5% of claudicators experience limb loss over a 5-year period.

In the case of resting ischemia there is a much more immediate threat of limb loss. Early management should include consultation with a vascular surgeon or other vascular specialist. Patients with rest pain and no open lesions can be managed initially with conservative protective measures, skin moisturizers, hygiene, posturing of the bed in reverse Trendelenberg (foot down) position, use of sheepskin or foam rubber under the feet as well as a foot board to elevate sheets and blankets off the toes. Podiatric consultation and support may be very helpful. If open lesions are present, these initial measures should be supplemented with topical antibiotic ointment and dressings, in conjunction with oral or intravenous antibiotics if there is evidence of infection involving the surrounding tissue. If there is swelling, purulence or fever, such lesions may need urgent surgical drainage to control infection.

In the great majority of patients with resting ischemia, it is critically important to establish improved circulation. Arterial imaging must precede revascularization, usually using contrast arteriography or MRI. Modern digital techniques have made arteriography relatively safe and comfortable. MRI is an adequate substitute for arteriography in many situations, and is particularly useful in patients with allergy or increased risk of renal dysfunction related to arteriographic contrast dye. Percutaneous therapy of appropriate iliac artery lesions using balloon angioplasty and stents is associated with complications in < 1% of patients and may be expected to produce a cumulative 5-year patency rate of 85–90%. Catheter-based therapy of the superficial femoral artery is similarly safe, though with somewhat less durable 5-year cumulative patency of about 60% under the best circumstances. These percutaneous methods can be repeated in many instances should the need arise.

A number of surgical options are available for treatment of high-grade or diffuse aortoiliac disease, tailoring the surgical procedure to the patient's needs and associated risk factors. In general, procedural mortality following surgery for aortoiliac disease is < 3%, with 5-year cumulative patency rates close to 90% for aortofemoral, iliofemoral and femorofemoral bypass. Long-term patency rates for axillofemoral bypass are not quite as favorable, averaging 75–80% in most series. Reconstructions below the groin are associated with roughly 2% operative mortality risk. Five year cumulative success rates are 80–85% for patients with claudication and 65–70% for patients with resting ischemia. Following revascularization, major amputation is necessary in less than 10% of patients within 5 years of intervention.

Venous disease
Acute deep vein thrombosis
Presentation
In many patients who present with DVT there is a history of predisposing risk factors including previous DVT, specific hypercoagulable states, pregnancy, malignancy or events such as a prolonged recumbency during travel, injury to the leg, hospitalization or recent surgery. Leg pain from DVT may first be noticeable upon arising after a night's rest or a long trip, or may have a more insidious onset. In general, the pain is constant and aching in quality, located in the muscle compartment surrounding and distal to the obstruction, with an element of sharpness referable to the involved vein segments. The patient will generally report aggravation of the pain with walking and dependency and some relief with elevation of the limb. Swelling is often reported and cyanosis from venous congestion may have been noticed. With complete ileofemoral obstruction resulting in *Phlegmasia alba dolens* and subsequent *Phlegmasia cerulea dolens*, pain will evolve into neuropathic numbness and paralysis as actual tissue ischemia supervenes on the basis of absence of sufficient venous outflow from the limb (Figure 6.6).

On inspection, swelling of the lower extremity may be evident, with an element of cyanosis and plethora. The swollen and involved portions of the leg will be tense and tender on the basis of venous inflammation and increased compartment pressure. Low-grade fever may be present. Flexion of the ankle may produce discomfort in the calf in the case of calf thrombosis (Homans' sign), though this finding is non-specific. An enhanced pattern of superficial venous channels may indicate presence of collaterals stimulated by obstruction of the deeper proximal veins. Elevation of the abnormal limb in tandem with the normal limb may demonstrate persistent filling of the superficial foot veins in the obstructed leg at a level when the normal leg veins have emptied. In extreme cases of ileofemoral thrombosis, the limb may have reduced arterial pulses or be pulseless, with evidence of sluggish flow in the toes and forefoot with impending capillary stasis and infarction of tissue.

It is important to recall that the clinical presentation of acute venous occlusion is notoriously non-specific, and that many patients experience significant venous thrombosis with no signs or symptoms whatsoever. Most prominent in the differential diagnosis are the postphlebitic syndrome, superficial thrombophlebitis, cellulitis and muscle or ligamentous injury.

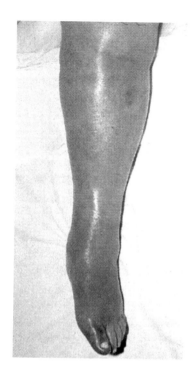

Figure 6.6 *Phlegmasia cerulea dolens* resulting from extensive acute ileofemoral vein thrombosis. Note swelling and cyanosis with congestive stasis of flow in toes causing necrosis. Adapted from Walker WF. *Color Atlas of Peripheral Vascular Diseases*. Copyright 1980, p. 94, with permission from Elsevier.

Laboratory

The most accurate means of differentiating DVT from other conditions is duplex ultrasound. Ultrasound performed in an experienced laboratory can identify both anatomic obstruction and physiological changes in flow with over 90% accuracy in veins proximal to the calf. Calf veins are also often visible, though with a somewhat higher incidence of inaccuracy. Though not routinely imaged in most peripheral vascular laboratories, the iliac veins and inferior vena cava may be interrogated indirectly by characterization of ultrasound flow patterns at the femoral level. Impedance plethysmography, pneumoplethysmography and phleborheography are less available but useful indirect means of identifying significant proximal venous obstruction. MRI may also be helpful, as may contrast venography, although both of these modalities are relatively expensive and unpleasant and add little to the initial diagnostic evaluation. All modalities are confounded to variable extents by the differential between acute thrombus and old postphlebitic changes in the vein.

A sizable minority of patients with venous thrombosis have a hypercoagulable state for which anticoagulation may be best prolonged. Laboratory assays should be performed for antiphospholipid syndrome, activated protein C resistance (factor V Leiden) and prothrombin G20210A mutant.

Management

Early management consists of prompt presumptive diagnosis followed by bed rest with leg elevation above the level of the heart. Confirmatory duplex ultrasound should be performed in conjunction with anticoagulation using intravenous unfractionated heparin or subcutaneous low-molecular-weight heparin in order to halt the process of thrombosis and enhance the natural fibrinolytic cascade which will result in partial or complete recanalization of the vein in the great majority of patients. Ordinarily, bed rest with elevation and heparin will result in improvement in symptoms due to decrease in swelling and inflammation and increase in collateral. Intravenous heparin or subcutaneous low-molecular-weight heparin should be continued until coumadin, which may be initiated on day 2 or 3, has resulted in elevation of prothrombin time and international normalized ratio (INR) to 18–20 s and 2.5–3.0, respectively. Mobilization of the patient is usually appropriate when the pain and swelling are sufficiently improved. Consultation with a vascular or hematology specialist may be appropriate should there be unusual circumstances such as phlegmasia, failure to respond, evidence of pulmonary embolus or difficulty with persistent symptoms. Selected patients may be treated with surgical thrombectomy or percutaneous suction thrombectomy and fibrinolysis. In general, inferior vena caval filters are not indicated unless there is a firm contraindication to anticoagulation or evidence of pulmonary embolus while adequately anticoagulated.

Superficial thrombophlebitis

Superficial thrombophlebitis involves branches of the veins in the subcutaneous tissue. Though sometimes associated with systemic disease, classically malignancy (Trousseau's syndrome), superficial phlebitis is more common among patients with a recent injury at the site of a superficial vein or with pre-existing varicose veins. A particularly bothersome time for superficial phlebitis is during the later stages of pregnancy. A minority of patients with superficial phlebitis have systemic hypercoagulable states.

The typical history is abrupt onset of sharply focused pain located in a linear pattern in the general distribution of the superficial venous trunks such as the greater saphenous or lesser saphenous vein. The region is indurated, red, very tender and surrounded by local subcutaneous swelling. There may be more than one focus of inflammation or evidence of previous burned out episodes from chronic hyperpigmentation and induration. Varicose veins are often present. In a minority, phlebitis may also involve the deep veins, either by direct extension or as part of a more generalized illness involving two sites simultaneously.

Superficial phlebitis is a non-bacterial sterile process. The most common alternative diagnoses in the differential are soft tissue cellulitis and traumatic contusion. Septic thrombophlebitis occurs rarely and usually is related to intravenous access involving the upper extremity. Presence of a history of venipuncture or drug abuse, high fever, diffuse linear pattern along the course of the vein and purulent drainage from a venipuncture site make septic phlebitis highly suspect.

Laboratory

The diagnosis of superficial phlebitis is nearly always clear enough on clinical grounds to make confirmatory laboratory study unnecessary. Nonetheless, duplex ultrasound can confirm phlebitis in a superficial vein and exclude concurrent involvement of the deep veins. Ultrasound is most valuable among patients with superficial phlebitis near the popliteal space or saphenofemoral junction in whom contiguous deep veins may be involved.

Management

A review of the patient's general health is important to exclude an underlying predisposing condition such as malignancy. Superficial phlebitis is best managed with non-steroidal anti-inflammatory medications such as indomethacin (25–50 mg tid) together with rest and elevation. Topical heat may help the symptoms. There is no role for antibiotics. The clinical picture should be followed closely to be certain that there is improvement rather than extension of the process. Should there be no improvement, increased doses of non-steroidals or intravenous heparin may be necessary. In selected resistant cases, superficial phlebitis may be treated by surgical excision of the involved vein. Care of pregnant patients must be coordinated with the involved obstetrician.

Chronic deep venous insufficiency

Presentation

Chronic obstruction or valvular incompetence of the deep veins is most commonly manifest as the postplebitic syndrome resulting from previous DVT, at times undocumented. A sizable minority of patients with deep venous insufficiency have primary valvular incompetence unrelated to DVT. The pain is typically located at the distal portion of the leg near the calf and ankle and consists of heaviness, tightness or pressure within the muscle compartments. It is aggravated by dependency and relieved by elevation. There is often associated swelling, varicose veins, and hyperpigmentation in the skin. Over time, eczema and ultimately ulceration with cellulitis supervene around the medial portion of the ankle just above the malleolus. In the small number of patients with chronic venous obstruction at a proximal level, swelling may be more prominent. Venous claudication may occur with such proximal obstruction, with a tightness and bursting sensation which is relieved after cessation of exercise as the leg empties via venous collaterals.

Examination may be completely normal, but most often a pattern of mild swelling over the ankle, varicosities, hyperpigmentation ('brawny induration') in the skin of the distal calf and ankle with a medial preponderance indicate the presence of longstanding deep venous insufficiency. Eczema and weeping or overt ulceration with surrounding cellulitis may be present (Figure 6.7).

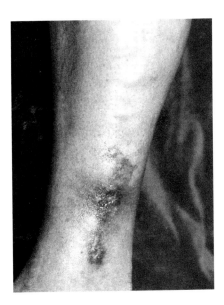

Figure 6.7 Chronic venous insufficiency with edema, varicose veins and hyperpigmentation with eczema and ulceration concentrated at medial ankle in region of perforator veins. Reprinted with permission from Altenkamper H, Eldenburg M. *Farbatlas der Phlebologie.* Hannover: Schlütersche, 1993.

Laboratory non-invasive study by duplex ultrasound provides valuable confirmation of the presence of deep venous scarring, obstruction or valvular incompetence. A baseline examination is generally valuable for later comparison in the event of the need for differentiation between chronic stable postphlebitic syndrome and superimposed acute DVT. Further anatomic study using MRI or venography may be appropriate should surgical intervention be recommended after consultation.

Early management
Symptomatic relief is generally provided by a combination of frequent limb elevation and external elastic compression by means of knee length ace bandage or 30–40 mmHg graduated compression support stockings. Antibiotics, possibly by intravenous route in severe cases, are important in the presence of inflammation with or without ulceration. Intermittent gauze dressings with wet to dry saline or an occlusive dressing using one of a variety of available products can reduce pain and exudate and foster healing of eczema and ulcers. The Unna paste boot is a reliable option which provides both topical dressing and support to the leg while assuring patient compliance and convenience. Early consultation with an appropriate specialist is usually indicated when ulceration is present. Life-long knee length elastic support is a prerequisite for successful management.

Chronic superficial venous disease
Presentation
Varicose enlargement of the superficial veins (greater saphenous and lesser saphenous) presents as a syndrome of localized heaviness and aching after

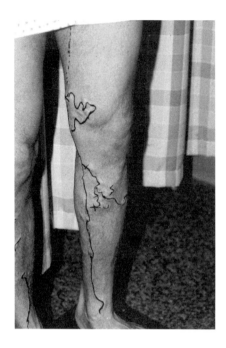

Figure 6.8 Primary varicose veins with involved greater saphenous vein and branches outlined with skin marker.

prolonged standing. Elevation or external elastic support generally provides relief. A localized injury may result in superficial phlebitis. A few patients with extraordinarily superficial thin-walled tributaries may experience painless bleeding from the varicosities. Patients with secondary varicose veins will generally have a history of associated deep venous insufficiency and previous DVT. In the case of primary varicose veins, most patients present in their third or fourth decades and have a family history of varicose veins. The veins follow a course of gradual progression, greatly exacerbated by pregnancies in the case of females.

Examination is best performed with the patient standing (Figure 6.8). The varicosities are most prominent distal to the knee where branches are larger and more superficial. There may be some focal areas of hyperpigmenation over the shin and medial ankle. Swelling is generally absent or mild unless there is deep venous involvement. The source of filling of the varicose system can be demonstrated by Trendelenberg test (Figure 6.9). The leg is elevated to empty the veins and a tourniquet is applied to prevent refilling of the vein from a superficial source when the leg is returned to a dependent position. If such refilling occurs despite the tourniquet, it must be via an incompetent perforator resulting from deep vein disease.

Because physical findings are usually obvious, laboratory has a limited role in confirming the diagnosis of superficial venous disease. In cases where the history and physical suggest that the varicosities are secondary rather than primary, duplex ultrasound may help characterize the deep venous

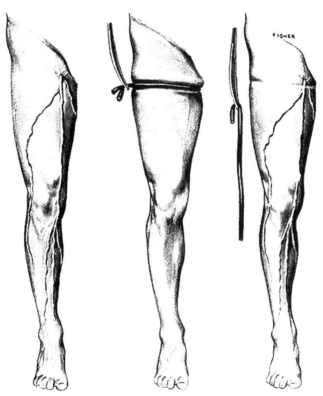

Figure 6.9 Trendelenberg test for assessing source of reflux into varicose veins. Varicosities are most pronounced with leg dependency (left). After elevation above head, a tourniquet is applied in proximal thigh to occlude superficial veins but not deep veins. If the varicosities are unfilled with dependency and tourniquet, the source of filling is superficial, most commonly the greater saphenous trunk (center). Rapid refilling of the varicosities with release of tourniquet confirms flow abnormality (right). Reprinted from Dodd H, Cockett FB. *The Pathology and Surgery of the Veins of the Lower Limb*, 2nd edn. Copyright 1976, p. 82, with permission from Elsevier.

abnormalities and identify any important perforating veins filling the superficial varicosities.

Management

Early therapy consists of reassurance with respect to any particular threat of blood clots or limb jeopardy. Support garments of a sensible nature such as pantyhose or leotards may completely relieve symptoms. With sufficient symptomatology, consultation may be appropriate, particularly in younger individuals in whom the problem usually progresses with time. If veins are relatively isolated and small, injection sclerotherapy or laser ablation may be helpful. Larger varicosities related to one of the saphenous trunks are generally best treated with surgery to ligate and remove ('strip') the veins.

Suggested reading

Creager MA, O'Leary DH, Doubilet PM. Noninvasive vascular testing In: Loscalzo J, Creager MA, Dzau VJ, eds. *Vascular Medicine,* 2nd edn. Boston: Little, Brown and Co., 1996; 415–444.

Dodd H, Cockett FB. *The Pathology and Surgery of the Veins of the Lower Limb.* Edinburgh: Livingstone, 1972.

Donaldson MC. Chronic venous disorders. In: Loscalzo J, Creager MA, Dzau VJ, eds. *Vascular Medicine,* 2nd edn. Boston: Little, Brown and Co., 1996; 1081–1102.

Gloviczki P. Venous disease: an overview. In: Rutherford RB, ed. *Vascular Surgery,* 5th edn. Philadelphia: W.B. Saunders Co., 2000; 1907–1919.

Kempczinski RP. The chronically ischemic leg: an overview. In: Rutherford RB, ed. *Vascular Surgery,* 5th edn. Philadelphia: W.B. Saunders Co., 2000; 917–927.

Ouriel K. Acute limb ischemia. In: Rutherford RB, ed. *Vascular Surgery,* 5th edn. Philadelphia: W.B. Saunders Co., 2000; 813–821.

Rutherford RB. Initial patient evaluation: the vascular consultation. In: Rutherford RB, ed. *Vascular Surgery,* 5th edn. Philadelphia: W.B. Saunders Co., 2000; 1–12.

Walker WF. *Color Atlas of Peripheral Vascular Diseases.* Chicago: Year Book Medical Publishers, 1980.

CHAPTER 7

Neuropathic leg pain

David C. Preston

Patients with disorders of the peripheral nervous system (mononeuropathy, polyneuropathy, plexopathy or radiculopathy) often present with the chief complaint of pain in one or both legs. Of course, leg pain of vascular and orthopedic etiology is ultimately perceived via the peripheral nervous system and may share many attributes of pain derived from primary disease of the nerves. The goal for the clinician is to be able to recognize primary neuropathic pain and separate it from the many secondary causes. The differential diagnosis, subsequent evaluation, and potential treatments are markedly different from disorders affecting blood vessels, bone, joints, and soft tissues. The situation is confounded by some disorders having a propensity to affect not only nerve but blood vessels and occasionally joints as well. Diabetes mellitus, with its frequent complication of peripheral neuropathy and association with peripheral vascular disease, is the most common condition in which differentiating the source of leg pain is difficult. However, with close attention to history, physical examination, and judicious use of laboratory testing, often the separation can be made, or at a minimum, an appreciation can be reached of how much each is contributing to the leg pain.

Anatomy of neuropathic pain

To understand neuropathic pain first requires some knowledge of the gross and microscopic anatomy of peripheral nerve. Peripheral nerve contains somatic and autonomic, motor and sensory fibers. All somatic motor fibers are ultimately derived from motor neurons that reside in the anterior gray matter of the spinal cord. Motor neurons receive direct information from the frontal lobe of the brain via the cortical spinal track (the upper motor neuron), as well as from numerous other indirect pathways connecting to adjacent spinal cord segments, the brain stem, the basal ganglia and the cerebral cortex. Autonomic motor fibers to the leg originate from cells in the intermediolateral gray matter of the spinal cord. They exit ventrally with the somatic motor fibers and run in the ventral (motor) roots.

On the sensory side, the primary sensory neuron is the dorsal root ganglion that, in contrast to the motor neuron, does not lie within the substance of the spinal cord, but resides outside in the intervertebral foramen of the spinal column. This cell is a bipolar cell giving rise to both a central and a peripheral process. The central processes of the dorsal root ganglia form the dorsal root entering the dorsal horn of the spinal cord, where some fibers ascend in the posterior columns of the spinal cord (supplying vibration and position sense), where others synapse, cross and then ascend in the contralateral anterior lateral spinothalamic track conveying pain and temperature. It is dysfunction or disease of this latter tract and its peripheral connections that are responsible for the perception of pain in the leg. The peripheral processes of the dorsal ganglion cell unite with the motor roots from the motor neurons of each spinal segment to form the spinal nerve. The spinal nerve exits through the intervertebral foramen (where it is susceptible to compression from disk herniation, spondylosis, etc.) and quickly bifurcates into a dorsal and ventral ramus. The dorsal and ventral rami both contain motor and sensory fibers. The dorsal rami supply the paraspinal muscles for motor function and the area over the skin of the back for sensation. The ventral rami in the lumbosacral region come together to form the lumbosacral plexus. From the lumbosacral plexus, individual peripheral nerves of the leg are derived. The major peripheral nerves of the leg are the femoral, sciatic (terminates into the tibial and common peroneal), superior gluteal, inferior gluteal, lateral cutaneous nerve of the thigh, and the posterior cutaneous nerve of the thigh.

Each peripheral nerve contains motor and sensory innervation from several spinal segments (myotomes and dermatomes, respectively). Nerve fibers ultimately supply all muscles for locomotion as well as sensory fibers to all skin areas for cutaneous sensation. In addition, there are sensory fibers to deep tissues including muscles, bones and joints, and autonomic fibers supplying blood vessels and sweat glands.

Microscopically, peripheral nerve contains both myelinated and unmyelinated nerve fibers. Myelin is derived from concentric rolls of Schwann cell cytoplasm (the Schwann cell being the major supporting cell of the peripheral nerve). Myelin is an effective insulator of peripheral nerve that greatly allows for dramatically increased speed of conduction compared with unmyelinated fibers (50 m/s compared with 1 m/s). Larger fibers have more myelin than smaller fibers and many small axons are not myelinated at all. The large myelinated fibers convey all motor function as well as sensory function for touch, vibration and joint position sense. The smaller axons, both myelinated and unmyelinated, supply pain and temperature sensation as well as autonomic function. It is disease or dysfunction of these small fibers that account for much of the pain and unpleasant dysesthesias associated with neuropathy and other disorders of the peripheral nervous system.

Internal anatomy of peripheral nerve is comparable to the internal anatomy of muscle. There are several layers of connective tissue (Figure 7.1). Around a nerve trunk is the thick epineurium, which at the nerve root level is a direct continuation of the dura mater. Beyond the epineurium, nerve fibers are grouped together in clusters known as fascicles. Each fascicle has a connective tissue barrier, the perineurium. Within each fascicle is additional connective tissue running between the individual nerve fibers known as the endoneurium. The epineurium has a rich anastomotic network of arteries

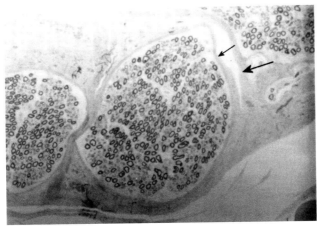

Figure 7.1 Internal peripheral nerve anatomy. Myelinated fibers are recognized as small dark rings (myelin) with a central clearing (axon). The endoneurium is present between axons. Axons are grouped into fascicles, surrounded by perineurium (small arrow). Surrounding the entire nerve is the last layer of connective tissue, the epineurium (large arrow). Reprinted with permission from Preston DC, Shapiro BE. *Electromyography and Neuromuscular Disorders*. Boston: Butterworth-Heinemann, 1998.

and veins known as the vasa nervosum. From this anastomotic network, individual venules and arterioles penetrate the peri- and endoneurium to supply the nerve.

Pathophysiology of neuropathic pain

When a nerve is injured, it can only react in a limited number of ways. Nerve dysfunction can cause either lack of function (negative symptoms and signs) or extra or disturbed function (positive symptoms and signs). When sensory fibers are diseased, extra or disturbed function is often more troubling than lack of function. Most can relate to leaning on an elbow, having the arm 'fall asleep' (lack of function—negative symptom) followed by return of blood flow leading to 'pins and needle' paresthesias (extra function—positive symptom). If motor nerve loses function, weakness, fatigue and atrophy develop. Extra or disturbed motor function may result in fasciculations or cramps. As for the sensory system, often the type of positive and negative symptoms denotes which type of nerve fiber has been affected. The large sensory nerve fibers convey touch, vibration and joint position sense. Lack of function of these fibers will lead to loss of these modalities on examination. Extra or disturbed function of this type of nerve will lead to 'pins and needle' paresthesias. This is in contrast to small fibers that convey pain and temperature which, when disordered, result in loss of temperature and pain sensation but, when disturbed or over-functioning, may cause burning, stinging, and other unpleasant paresthesias.

Most neuropathic pain occurs because of disturbed function or hyperactivity of the small pain fibers. Patients typically use the words 'burning', 'jabbing', or 'shooting' to describe these abnormal sensations. When these sensations are due to primary dysfunction of peripheral nerve, they are usually perceived as superficial, affecting the skin. Lightly touching the skin, even with non-painful stimuli, may lead to the generation of painful paresthesias. Such would not be expected in primary orthopedic or vascular diseases.

Mechanisms of nerve injury

Nerve can be injured by a variety of mechanisms. First, transient compression will result in ischemia to nerve that can quickly be reversed when the compression is lessened. No structural abnormality occurs. If the compression is more severe or lasts a greater length of time, subsequent mechanical deformation of the myelin sheath will occur, followed by frank demyelination. Although there is a structural abnormality of the myelin sheath, the underlying axon remains intact. If the compression is relieved, repair can occur by the process of remyelination that usually occurs over several weeks.

If the compression lasts long enough or is more severe, not only will there be mechanical deformation of myelin, but also of the underlying axon as well. Subsequently, the distal axon undergoes the process of wallerian degeneration which results in complete degeneration of the axon and its myelin sheath distal to the compression. This type of injury is much more serious than simple demyelination. If the compression is relieved, the nerve can recover, but must do so by regrowing from the terminal stump. If there has not been disruption of the connective tissue surrounding the nerve, the nerve will commonly be successful in regrowing. However, this regrowth is quite slow (typically the rate of slow axonal transport does not occur faster than a millimeter a day).

Finally, the most severe type of compressive or traumatic injury is one where there is not only disruption of the axon with its myelin sheath, but also of the surrounding connective tissue. In this type of injury, the nerve has been severely disrupted and any attempt at regrowth is usually futile. The nerve often grows into a tangled painful scar known as a neuroma.

Beyond compression and trauma, there are additional mechanisms which may damage nerve. The most common are various metabolic and toxic factors that may adversely poison the metabolic machinery of nerve. There are many endogenous (e.g. liver and renal disease) and exogenous toxins (e.g. alcohol, prescription drugs, chemotherapy, occupational toxins) that may damage peripheral nerve. Most of these toxic metabolic conditions tend to cause the most severe dysfunction to the nerves which are the longest. These nerves have the greatest metabolic demand and therefore are much more susceptible. Clinically, this results in the most distal and longest nerve being affected first (the longest nerve in the body is the sciatic nerve running from the back to the tip of the toes, approximately three feet in length).

Besides toxic and metabolic factors, there are several other mechanisms of nerve injury. Many inherited and genetic abnormalities may adversely affect either the motor neuron, its axon or the myelin sheath. Inherited neuropathies are often quite mild or advance slowly, over years or decades. Rarely, peripheral nerve may be damaged by frank infiltration of tumor of granulomatous tissue. Finally, there are many inflammatory (infectious, but more often, autoimmune) conditions which depending on the site of inflammation may damage the peripheral nerve. Lyme, leprosy, cytomegalovirus (CMV), herpes simplex virus (HSV), herpes zoster virus (HZV), and human immuno-deficiency virus (HIV) are among the various infectious agents that commonly affect peripheral nerve. Autoimmune attack on the myelin nerve sheath results in Guillain–Barré syndrome acutely and when chronic, chronic inflammatory demyelinating polyneuropathy (CIDP). Vasculitis, an inflammatory attack directed at blood vessels, may have profound secondary effects on nerve via ischemia and subsequent nerve infarction.

Clinical assessment

Recognition of peripheral nerve dysfunction involves a directed neurological history and examination with special emphasis on the motor and sensory system and reflexes. During the motor examination all major muscle groups in the lower extremity should be inspected for the presence of normal muscle bulk and fasciculations (involuntary brief muscle twitches). Decreased muscle bulk (atrophy) and fasciculations are signs of peripheral nerve disease. In addition, testing muscle tone (resistance to passive motion) of both legs is important. Increased muscle tone may be seen in disorders of the central nervous system (spinal cord or brain), but may sometimes be a manifestation of guarding due to pain. Muscle strength should be tested for dorsiflexion, plantarflexion, inversion and eversion around the ankle; flexion and extension around the knee; and flexion, extension, adduction and abduction around the hip. It is important to recognize that subtle weakness is often missed on the examining table. To demonstrate subtle weakness, it is often very useful to put patients through functional tests or put their muscles at mechanical disadvantage (toe and heel walking, walking up and down stairs, getting out of a low chair without using their hands, doing a deep knee bend, etc.).

The sensory examination should include assessment of vibration sense at the great toe, ankle and knee, both in comparison with the examiner and the contralateral asymptomatic leg if possible. In addition, joint position sense of the great toe and ankle should be assessed. Both vibration and joint position sense test large sensory fibers. To test small fiber function, 'pin-prick' and temperature should be assessed in both legs. It is important to check the distribution of all major nerves. Therefore as a rule it is important to check sensation in the webspace of the great toe (deep peroneal), dorsum of the foot (superficial peroneal), sole (tibial nerve), lateral calf (superficial peroneal), medial calf (saphenous), anterior thigh (femoral), lateral thigh (lateral femoral cutaneous nerve), and the posterior thigh (posterior cutaneous nerve of the thigh).

The reflex examination should be a routine part of any examination of a patient with a painful leg. Each reflex is mediated via a sensory afferent pathway, a synapse in the spinal cord, and a subsequent motor efferent. Both knee and ankle reflexes need to be compared and contrasted with each other. The knee reflex travels through the femoral nerve, lumbar plexus and L2–4 nerve roots. The ankle reflex travels through the tibial nerve, sciatic nerve, lumbosacral plexus and the S1–2 nerve roots. Reduced or absent reflexes are a sign of peripheral nerve disease. Bilaterally reduced ankle reflexes are common in polyneuropathy. Any significant reflex asymmetry suggests a focal nerve lesion somewhere along the reflex arc. The Babinski response should be elicited by stroking the lateral sole and looking for a normal flexion movement of the great toe. An extensor response suggests the presence of a central nervous system lesion.

Finally, the extremities should be inspected for trophic changes. Many of these changes may be seen in vascular disease as well, including change in the color of the skin, loss of hair and shininess of the skin. Ultimately, all autonomic function is mediated via the peripheral nerves. As autonomic fibers innervate blood vessels, dysfunction of these fibers can result in vascular changes, usually most marked distally at the small artery or arteriole level. Autonomic fibers are mediated by small myelinated and unmyelinated nerve fibers, the same as fibers that mediate pain and temperature sensation. Some neuropathies will preferentially affect small fibers (e.g. amyloid, alcohol, diabetes) leading both to distal autonomic and pain/temperature dysfunction.

In a patient with a painful leg or legs, any definite abnormality of the motor, sensory or reflex examination suggests, at a minimum, that there may be a possible neurological component to the patient's pain. As the differential diagnosis of peripheral nerve disorders is quite large, the possibilities must first be limited by the neuroanatomic localization. Only certain disorders affect certain parts of the peripheral nervous system. Some symptoms of polyneuropathy, sciatic neuropathy and lumbar radiculopathy may be very similar, but the differential diagnosis of disorders affecting those three sites is very different. The pattern of weakness, atrophy, reflex loss and sensory disturbance usually allows a correct neuroanatomic localization. Often, the localization is confirmed or defined by nerve conduction studies and electromyography. With the anatomy localized, in conjunction with the history, the differential diagnosis quickly narrows and allows a more directed and appropriate evaluation.

Disease of the nerve root

Radiculopathy
Diseases of the nerve roots are among the most common afflictions of man. Each nerve root contains sensory and motor fibers supplying a specific area of

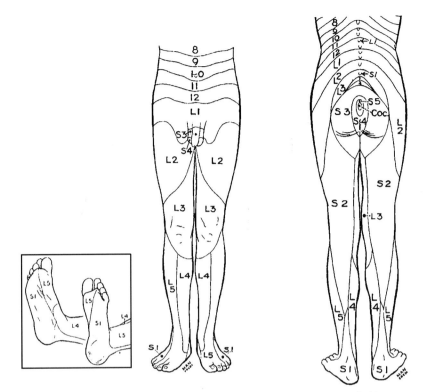

Figure 7.2 Lower extremity dermatome. A dermatome is the cutaneous area supplied from one spinal segment (i.e. one sensory nerve root). Despite the apparent simplicity of dermatomal charts, in actuality there is a wide overlap of adjacent dermatomes. Consequently, a nerve root lesion, even if severe, never results in anesthesia, but only altered or decreased sensation. Reprinted from Haymaker W, Woodhal B. *Peripheral Nerve Injuries*. Copyright 1945, with permission from Elsevier.

skin (dermatome) (Figure 7.2), and a specific number of muscles (myotome). However, any particular area of skin may receive innervation from several overlapping dermatomes, and all muscles receive innervation from more than one myotome. Accordingly, with disease of a single nerve root, dense sensory loss does not develop. Patients with radiculopathy who complain of sensory symptoms in one dermatome more often have vague and ill-defined sensory loss on examination (due to the wide overlap of adjacent dermatomes).

Likewise, dysfunction of one nerve root never leads to paralysis but only to weakness. For instance, the quadriceps is innervated by L2–L4 nerve roots via the femoral nerve. A severe lesion of the femoral nerve will result in severe weakness of the quadriceps (the quadriceps are only innervated by the femoral nerve). However, any equally severe L4 radiculopathy will result in only mild to moderate weakness of the quadriceps. Paralysis does not develop due to the contribution of L2 and L3.

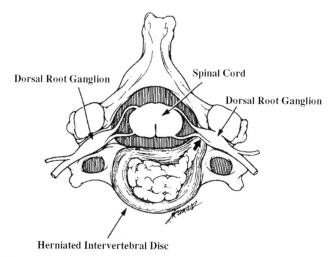

Figure 7.3 Radiculopathy secondary to a herniated intervertebral disc. Herniated discs are most often lateral and posterior, which compress the exiting nerve root. Reprinted with permission from Wilbourn AJ. In Brown WF, Bolton CF, eds. *Clinical Electromyography*, 2nd edn. Boston: Butterworth-Heinemann, 1993.

Radiculopathy is usually caused by compression as the nerve root leaves the intervertebral foramen (Figure 7.3). This most often results from a herniated intervertebral disc (especially in younger individuals) or as a result of hypertrophy of bone or ligaments in older individuals (i.e. spondylosis). By far the most common sites for disc herniation are at L4–5 with compression of the L5 nerve root and at L5–S1 with compression of the S1 root. In addition, radiculopathy may result from other mass lesions, including metastatic diseases of the spine, or rarely abscess within the epidural space. In the two latter conditions, radiculopathy usually occurs prior to frank spinal cord compression.

Radiculopathy is the most common source of neuropathic pain in the leg. Though the lesion is at the nerve root level, pain is often referred into the leg in a radiating manner in the distribution of the nerve root. However, the majority of the pain is proximal, usually in the back, buttocks, and upper thigh. Upper lumbar radiculopathies (L2–4) may refer pain anteriorly into the thigh whereas lower lumbosacral (L5–S1) radiculopathies refer pain posterior and lateral, generally to a level below the knee. Patients characteristically find prolonged sitting and standing difficult. Coughing and sneezing can exacerbate the radiating pain down the leg. This occurs as coughing and sneezing both increase intraspinal pressure. Simple movement or manipulation of the back is painful. Patients often find that the most comfortable position is lying on their side with their hips and knees in a flexed posture.

Radiculopathy should be suspected in any patient with leg pain who also has coexistent back pain with radiation of that pain down the leg. Pain from

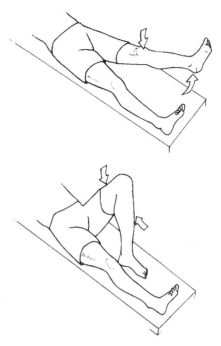

Figure 7.4 The classic straight leg raise test consists of two parts: a straight leg raise followed by a second lift with knee flexed. The first should cause radiating pain (not merely tightness in the posterior thigh), the latter should not. Reprinted with permission from Hlavin ML, Hardy RW Jr. Lumbar disc disease. *Neurosurg Q* 1991; **1**:29.

the ligaments and joints of the back and hip may radiate into the proximal lower extremity but not below the knee. Mechanical movements that increase the pain such as bending or straightening the leg also suggest the presence of radiculopathy, and there are a number of tests that rely on this principle, including straight leg raising and the 'bowstring' sign (Figure 7.4). The level of radiculopathy can often be deduced by the distribution of muscle weakness, which reflexes are depressed or in what areas the patient reports altered or disturbed sensation. The important clinical findings in lumbosacral radiculopathy at different levels are outlined in Table 7.1.

Polyradiculopathy

Beyond an isolated radiculopathy, root disease may manifest by many or all the lumbosacral nerve roots being affected at the same time (lumbosacral polyradiculopathy). This can occur in several situations. The first is the cauda equina syndrome, which can occur either acutely or chronically. Anatomically, the spinal cord ends at the L1 vertebra with the lumbosacral nerve roots running caudally through the thecal sac before exiting at their appropriate level (grossly, these nerve roots resemble a horse's tail, hence, cauda equina). Compression of the cauda equina may occur acutely as a result of either massive disc herniation or hemorrhage; it may occur gradually with tumor affecting all the lumbosacral nerve routes. In the acute syndrome, the patient

Table 7.1 Common lumbar radiculopathies.

Root	Pain location	Sensory disturbance	Weakness	Reflex change
L3	Anterior thigh, groin	Anterior thigh	Iliopsoas, hip adductors, quadriceps	Knee
L4	Anterior thigh	Medial calf, anterior thigh	Quadriceps, hip adductors, tibialis anterior	Knee
L5	Posterolateral thigh and calf, extending into great toe and dorsum foot	Dorsum foot, great toe, lateral calf	Tibialis posterior, extensor hallicus longus, hip abductors, tibialis anterior	None
S1	Posterolateral thigh and calf, extending into lateral toes and sole	Lateral foot, posterior calf, sole	Gastrocnemius, toe flexors, hip extension	Ankle

Modified from Geckle DS, Hlavin MI. Spondylosis and disc disease. In Samuels MA, Feske S, eds. *Office Practice of Neurology*, New York: Churchill-Livingstone, 1995.

develops significant back pain, a rapidly progressive paralysis of both legs, numbness of both legs including the genital and anal regions (the sacral dermatomes), and bladder and bowel dysfunction. An acute cauda equina syndrome is a neurological emergency requiring urgent imaging of the lower spine to exclude a compressive lesion which may require surgical decompression. Rarely an acute cauda equina syndrome may develop with a normal computed tomography (CT) or magnetic resonance imaging (MRI). These are the result of infiltration by tumor or granulomatous tissue, or more often from infection, especially HSV and CMV viruses. CMV has a predilection to cause this syndrome in immunosuppressed patients, especially those with HIV.

The other situation in which a lumbosacral polyradiculopathy can occur is the condition of spinal stenosis or neurogenic claudication. Spinal stenosis is a degenerative disease of the lumbosacral spine which usually occurs in older individuals from a combination of degenerative joint disease, ligament and joint facet hypertrophy, abnormal bone formation, and disc bulging/herniation resulting effectively in decreased space in the thecal sac. The nerve roots initially are intermittently compressed when the patient assumes the standing position. Patients give a clear history of pain that develops in the back with radiation into the buttocks and legs with walking. The pain is relieved by rest and often suggests the diagnosis of vascular claudication. The key to separating neurogenic claudication from the more typical vascular claudication is that neurogenic claudication requires that the patient sit for the pain to go away. This is in contrast to the patient with vascular claudication, who can simply rest in a standing posture. In addition, patients with neurogenic claudication often develop some cutaneous sensory symptoms or paresthesias suggesting that their abnormality involves nerve.

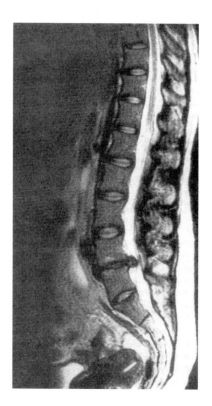

Figure 7.5 Lumbosacral disc herniation causing nerve root compression. Sagittal, T2 weighted magnetic resonance image of the lumbosacral spine showing a large herniated disc at the L4–5 level. Reprinted with permission from Katirji B, Shapiro B, Kaminski H *et al.*, eds. *Neuromuscular Disorders in Clinical Practice*. Boston: Butterworth-Heinemann, 2002.

Evaluation of radiculopathy/polyradiculopathy

If the history and physical examination suggest a progressive radiculopathy or polyradiculopathy, then further laboratory and radiological investigation is required.

The evaluation of a patient with a suspected radiculopathy or polyradiculopathy involves imaging of the back, selective nerve conduction studies/EMG, and in some cases, cerebrospinal fluid (CSF) examination. Imaging with CT myelogram or MRI scans can usually identify the presence of a structural lesion entrapping the nerve roots (disc herniation, spinal stenosis, abscess, tumor, or spinal cord malformation) (Figure 7.5). MRI is the most sensitive and useful test to obtain in this setting, and should be obtained urgently if the symptom complex has occurred over hours or days.

It is important to note that radiculopathy and polyradiculopathy may both occur without a structural lesion seen on MRI or CT myelogram. In these cases (suspected radiculopathy clinically, but with normal imaging), further investigation is required, usually with nerve conduction studies/EMG and CSF examination.

Non-mechanical radiculopathy can occur secondarily to nerve infarction (e.g. vasculitis, diabetes) or nerve infiltration (e.g. granulomatous disease such as sarcoid or from direct invasion by malignancy). Several infectious agents can directly infect nerve or cause a secondary inflammation. Infections which can affect the nerve roots include Lyme disease, Herpes Zoster, CMV, HSV, HIV, as well as rare cases of tuberculosis and fungi. Abnormal CSF studies will be found in most of these conditions.

Nerve conduction studies and EMG are often useful in patients with suspected radiculopathy. Nerve conduction and EMG can aid with the localization of the neurological lesion, usually differentiating a nerve root lesion from a peripheral nerve or lumbosacral plexus lesion. However, the EMG may remain normal up to 2 weeks after compression. Often, it is quite difficult to differentiate clinically a lumbosacral plexus lesion from a lumbosacral radiculopathy (another cause of normal imaging). EMG is often useful in making the differentiation between root and plexus disease. Electrical studies also add information about the function of the nerve root. A radiculopathy, severe enough to cause some wallerian degeneration, will result in denervation of the muscle fibers which can be easily seen on EMG.

Therapy of radiculopathy/polyradiculopathy

Therapy is tailored to the type of lesion and the amount of neurological disability. Many cases of disc herniation can be treated conservatively with bed rest and analgesics followed by gentle mobilization and later physical therapy. This should be the first approach unless there is a bowel, bladder or motor deficit on testing. The long-term goal is to reduce pressure on the lumbar spine by a combination of weight loss, proper posture, and an exercise program to increase the strength of the back and abdominal musculature. Indications for surgery usually include lack of improvement with conservative therapy, patient preference or a significant or progressive neurological deficit. There are many surgical procedures now for disc herniation including microscopic discectomy and endoscopic discectomy.

In case of mass lesions other than disc herniation, surgery is usually indicated. Compression by tumor may be treated with steroids and radiation if the tumor source is already known and characterized. If not, surgery is needed not only for decompression, but for definitive diagnosis. Likewise, abscess is usually treated with surgical drainage, culture and systemic antibiotics.

Therapy for neurogenic claudication usually involves surgery as well. However, the timing of surgery needs to be individualized based on the disability of the patient. If the patient who is also a poor surgical candidate develops minor claudication after several blocks of walking, it is probably best to treat such a patient conservatively and to have the patient adjust their behavior accordingly. However, if a patient is otherwise a good surgical risk and the degree of disability is significantly interfering with the quality of the patient's life, then decompressive therapy is indicated.

Disease of the lumbosacral plexus

After exiting the intervertebral foramina, the lumbosacral nerve roots (L1–S3) come together to form the lumbosacral plexus. Disease of the lumbosacral plexus may present in a very similar manner to diseases of the nerve root and cause pain into the leg. Lumbosacral plexus lesions are usually divided anatomically into disease of the upper plexus (lumbar plexus) and of the lower plexus (lumbosacral plexus). Lumbar plexopathies affect predominantly the L2–L4 fibers resulting in weakness of the quadriceps, iliopsoas and thigh adductor muscles (femoral and obturator nerves). The knee jerk is frequently depressed. Pain develops in the pelvis with radiation into the anterior thigh. Sensory loss may be apparent over the anterior medial and lateral thigh as well as the medial part of the calf. Lesions of the lower lumbosacral plexus affect predominantly the L4–S2 nerve fibers. Patients typically describe a deep boring pain in the pelvis with radiation posteriorly in the thigh. Sometimes, the nerve fibers destined for the peroneal nerve will be preferentially affected with the patient presenting with foot drop and sensory disturbance over the dorsum of the foot and lateral calf. This pattern may be difficult to differentiate from an isolated lesion of the common peroneal nerve, unless electrodiagnostic studies are performed.

Akin to diseases of the nerve root, the etiology of lumbosacral plexopathy is divided into structural disease and non-structural disease. Structural disease includes local invasion by tumor, most typically bladder, uterine, ovarian, prostate or colon. In addition, a mass lesion may occur as a result of a retroperitoneal hemorrhage which commonly occurs in the substance of the psoas muscle. Such can occur as the result of an aortic aneurysm rupture or more commonly as a spontaneous occurrence in a patient who is anticoagulated. Lumbosacral plexopathy may also occur on a structural basis in women with endometriosis with implantation of abnormal tissue on the plexus.

In addition, several non-structural causes of lumbosacral plexopathy occur. This most commonly occurs in patients with diabetes mellitus. Known also as proximal diabetic neuropathy or plexopathy, diabetic amyotrophy classically affects the lumbar plexus. Patients may have either mild or longstanding diabetes. They present with severe deep boring pain in the pelvis or proximal thigh. Movement is often difficult. The pain may last for weeks. As the pain slowly dissipates, it becomes apparent that the patient also has significant weakness out of proportion to the pain. Diabetic amyotrophy commonly affects the femoral and obturator nerves with prominent wasting of the anterior medial thigh musculature. Knee reflexes are often absent on the involved side. Despite the prominent pain, atrophy and weakness, there is often very little sensory loss. Usually, patients who develop diabetic amyotrophy will also have coexistent diabetic polyneuropathy, and thus will have some sensory disturbance distal in their legs. Lumbosacral plexopathy can also occur on a non-structural basis from radiation damage, usually administered previously for the treatment of tumor. Radiation plexopathy is typically painless in comparison with direct infiltration of the plexus, which usually causes pain. Rare cases of idiopathic lumbosacral plexitis may occur similarly to brachial plexitis in the arm. This often occurs a week or two after an immunological inciting event such as a cold, flu or immunization. In some cases, there will be no clear inciting event. Patients develop severe deep pain along with clear neurological signs or symptoms. The pain often lasts for weeks or months with all imaging studies being unremarkable.

Evaluation of lumbosacral plexopathy

If the history and physical examination suggest a lumbosacral plexopathy, then further laboratory and radiological investigation is required. Of utmost importance is to exclude diabetes mellitus with a fasting blood sugar and hemoglobin A_{1c}. Next, most patients require imaging of the pelvis to exclude a mass lesion. Often, the back needs to be imaged as well, as symptoms and signs of lumbosacral radiculopathy may easily mimic plexopathy.

Nerve conduction studies and EMG are indicated in the evaluation of lumbosacral plexopathy. First, nerve conductions and EMG can often localize the lesion to the plexus and exclude mononeuropathies (e.g. femoral, sciatic) and radiculopathies which can mimic plexopathy. EMG may be normal in unusual lesions which only irritate nerve but do not result in any axonal loss. In the case of radiation damage to the lumbosacral plexus, the presence of myokymia on EMG is often diagnostic. Myokymia is the spontaneous grouped repetitive discharges of a motor nerve which is highly characteristic of radiation damage. In superficial muscles, myokymia can be recognized by an undulating, worm-like movement of muscle. However, myokymia is much more easily appreciated on EMG which can sample deeper muscles.

Therapy of lumbosacral plexopathy

Compressive lesions by tumor are treated in the usual way with chemotherapy and radiation. In patients with diabetic amyotrophy and idiopathic plexitis, the condition is usually self limited but may last many months. Some cases of idiopathic plexitis may respond to intravenous gamma globulin and other immunomodulating therapies. These treatments are best reserved for patients who continue to process for several months and do not improve spontaneously. Otherwise, therapy is directed at improving muscle function by strengthening and physical therapy. Pain is often difficult to treat. Treatment of neuropathic pain from plexopathy is similar to treatment of neuropathic pain from any cause (see below).

Disease of individual peripheral nerves

Other than diseases of the lumbosacral nerve roots and plexus, polyneuropathies and mononeuropathies can affect the leg. Polyneuropathy affects both legs, usually in a symmetrical manner. Polyneuropathy which involves the small sensory fibers usually results in distal pain and burning. Mononeuropathies affect only one nerve and thus only affect one leg at a time. Depending on the type of injury, mononeuropathy may also result in significant pain in the distribution of the nerve. The diagnosis of mononeuropathy

Table 7.2 Lower extremity mononeuropathies.

Nerve	Sensory disturbance	Weakness	Reflex change
Lateral cutaneous of the thigh	Lateral thigh	None	None
Posterior cutaneous of the thigh	Posterior thigh	None	None
Superior gluteal	None	Hip abduction and internal rotation	None
Inferior gluteal	None	Hip extension	None
Femoral	Anterior thigh, medial calf	Hip flexion, knee extension	Knee
Saphenous	Medial calf	None	None
Obturator	Medial thigh	Hip adduction	None
Sciatic	Sole, lateral and posterior calf, dorsal foot	Knee flexion, all ankle movements	Ankle
Peroneal	Lateral calf, dorsal foot	Ankle dorsiflexion and eversion	None
Tibial	Sole, posterior calf	Ankle plantarflexion and inversion	Ankle
Plantar	Sole	Intrinsic foot	None

is usually based on the pattern of weakness and numbness (Table 7.2). The more common neuropathies affecting the lower extremities are the following.

Lateral femoral cutaneous neuropathy ('*Meralgia paresthetica*')

The lateral femoral cutaneous nerve runs as a direct extension off the lumbar plexus, around the pelvic brim to pass under the inguinal ligament to supply an oval area of skin over the lateral thigh (Figure 7.6). Entrapment of the lateral femoral cutaneous nerve may occur under the inguinal ligament resulting in a painful burning patch in the anterior lateral thigh. This is known as *Meralgia paresthetica*. As the nerve supplies no muscle, there is no reflex loss, no muscle atrophy or weakness. Obesity, tight clothing and diabetes are risk factors for this entrapment neuropathy.

Femoral neuropathy

The femoral nerve is derived from the L2–L4 nerve roots. The femoral nerve first supplies the iliopsoas muscle before running under the inguinal ligament where it divides into motor and sensory branches. The motor fibers supply the sartorius and pectineus muscles and the four heads of the quadriceps femoris muscle. Sensory fibers branch into three divisions supplying the anterior medial thigh, intermediate thigh, and medial calf.

Isolated femoral neuropathy is rare. It most often occurs as the result of compression from traction or stretch during pelvic surgery. In addition, the femoral nerve can become entrapped under the inguinal ligament if the leg is maintained in a lithotomy position for a prolonged period, as often happens

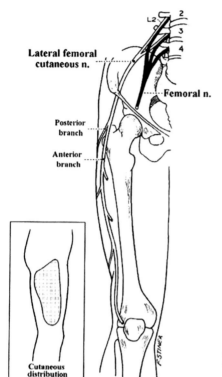

Lateral femoral
cutaneous n.

Femoral n.

Posterior
branch

Anterior
branch

Cutaneous
distribution

Figure 7.6 Anatomy of the lateral femoral cutaneous nerve. Adapted from Haymaker W, Woodhal B. *Peripheral Nerve Injuries*. Copyright 1945, with permission from Elsevier.

during pelvic surgery. Iatrogenic femoral neuropathy can occur in the inguinal region from misguided femoral catheterizations or subsequent to hematoma formation. Patients with femoral neuropathy develop buckling of their knee (due to quadriceps weakness), loss of the knee jerk, and sensory disturbance over the anterior thigh and medial calf.

Saphenous neuropathy

The saphenous nerve is the terminal extension of the femoral nerve supplying sensation to the medial calf. An isolated lesion of the saphenous nerve does not result in any motor weakness but only disturbed sensation over the medial calf (Figure 7.7). Although a saphenous neuropathy may be part of a larger femoral neuropathy, it may occur as an isolated finding as a result of trauma to the knee, or as an iatrogenic complication following orthopedic surgery at the knee or venous grafting for coronary artery bypass operations.

Tibial neuropathy

The tibial nerve is derived from the distal sciatic nerve above the popliteal fossa. The tibial nerve provides motor innervation to the muscles which plantarflex and invert the ankle as well as supplying most of the intrinsic foot

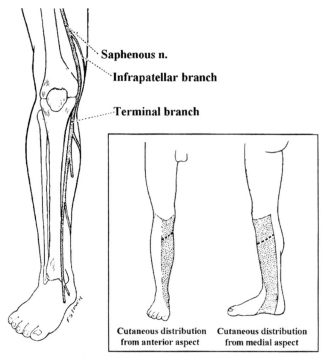

Saphenous n.

Infrapatellar branch

Terminal branch

Cutaneous distribution from anterior aspect   Cutaneous distribution from medial aspect

Figure 7.7 Anatomy of the saphenous nerve. Reprinted from Haymaker W, Woodhal B. *Peripheral Nerve Injuries*. Copyright 1945, with permission from Elsevier.

muscles. Tibial sensory fibers supply the lateral foot, posterior calf and the sole of the foot. Patients with tibial neuropathy will have difficulty walking and will be unable to walk on their tiptoes. The ankle jerk will be depressed or absent and sensation may be abnormal over the posterior calf, lateral foot, and sole. Isolated tibial neuropathies are uncommon; they may result from unusual mass lesion in the popliteal fossa (Baker's cyst, popliteal aneurysm, hemorrhage).

Peroneal neuropathy

The peroneal nerve, like the tibial nerve, is derived from the distal sciatic nerve in the popliteal fossa. The common peroneal nerve shortly bifurcates into the deep and superficial peroneal nerves. The deep peroneal nerve innervates the muscle which dorsiflexes the ankle and toes, and supplies sensation to the webspace between the great and second toe. The superficial peroneal nerve supplies muscles which evert the ankle as well as providing sensation to the lateral calf and dorsum of the foot. The peroneal nerve is vulnerable to injury and compression at the level of the fibular neck where it is quite superficial. Patients with peroneal neuropathy may develop pain about the lateral knee associated with foot drop and numbness over the lateral calf and dorsum of the foot.

Sciatic neuropathy

The sciatic nerve is the largest nerve in the body receiving nerve fibers from the L4–S3 nerve roots. The sciatic nerve leaves the pelvis under the piriformis muscle to supply the lateral and medial hamstrings before terminating in the peroneal and tibial nerves. Patients with sciatic neuropathy develop a combination of peroneal and tibial neuropathy in addition to weakness of hamstrings. All movement around the ankle will be weak or paralyzed. Sensory disturbance will develop over the lateral calf, dorsum and sole of the foot. The ankle jerk will commonly be absent. Acute sciatic neuropathies are usually the result of trauma, missile injury, prolonged immobilization, or infarction. Slowly progressive sciatic neuropathies often suggest slowly grow-ing mass lesions, usually a tumor.

Plantar neuropathy (tarsal tunnel syndrome)

The tibial nerve terminates in the medial ankle dividing into the medial and lateral plantar nerves and the calcaneal nerves. The plantar nerves supply the intrinsic foot musculature and sensation to the medial and lateral sole, respectively. As the nerve enters the foot, it runs under the flexor retinaculum on the medial ankle, known as the tarsal tunnel. Entrapment of the distal tibial in this tunnel results in local ankle pain with loss of sensation or neuropathic symptoms involving the sole of the foot.

Polyneuropathy

Polyneuropathies are probably the most common of all nerve lesions affecting the leg and usually present in a symmetric pattern, affecting both legs. Toxic, metabolic, and genetic polyneuropathies all present in a length-dependent fashion. The longest nerve, which carries the greatest metabolic demand, is the first to be affected. Accordingly, patients with polyneuropathy present with sensory disturbance on the soles of the feet which then slowly advances up the foot and into the ankle. Only when the level of sensory disturbance reaches the upper calf do patients start to develop sensory disturbance in their fingers (i.e. the stocking glove pattern). This occurs as the distance between the cervical spinal cord and the fingers is the same as between the lumbosacral spinal cord and the upper calf.

There are a vast number of conditions which can cause polyneuropathy. The differential diagnosis of polyneuropathy is often narrowed by knowing the following:

1 Tempo of the disease (acute, subacute, chronic, progressive or relapsing/remitting).

2 Fiber types involved (motor, sensory-large fiber, sensory-small fiber, autonomic).

3 Axonal or demyelinating or mixed (usually based on nerve conduction studies or biopsy).
4 Family history of polyneuropathy.
5 History of medical conditions often associated with polyneuropathy (diabetes, cancer, connective tissue disease, malnutrition, HIV infection).
6 Toxic exposure history (chemicals, medicines, alcohol).

Polyneuropathies are often associated with some degree of pain or unpleasant dysesthesias. However, several neuropathies predominantly affect small sensory fibers and are significantly associated with neuropathic pain. Patients present with distal burning and dysesthetic pain, and in some cases, distal autonomic changes in the foot and lower leg. Among these, the most common is the polyneuropathy associated with diabetes. Diabetes is the most common cause of neuropathy in North America and can affect peripheral nerve in a variety of ways: polyneuropathy, lumbosacral plexopathy, radiculopathy, and various mononeuropathies. Although diabetic polyneuropathy affects large sensory fibers as well, there is usually a distinct small-fiber component causing burning dysesthetic pain.

Several toxic and metabolic conditions (e.g. arsenic, thallium, thiamine deficiency) can result in a small-fiber polyneuropathy. Among them, the most common is polyneuropathy due to alcohol.

Inflammatory conditions may cause a painful neuropathy. Ischemia due to vasculitis often results in frank infarction of nerve. A patient may describe deep boring pain often at the infarction site followed by clear nerve dysfunction distally. In the leg, the sciatic nerve is most prone to nerve infarction in the proximal thigh, a watershed area for nerve ischemia. In contrast to nearly all polyneuropathies, vasculitic polyneuropathy usually presents in an asymmetrical pattern. Individual nerves are infarcted in a step-wise manner (i.e. the mononeuritis multiplex pattern). Over time, a confluent pattern develops that can be difficult to differentiate from the common stocking glove pattern. Other than vasculitis, polyneuropathy may occur from ischemia of other causes. Compartment syndromes, if not treated acutely, result in both nerve and muscle ischemia associated with significant pain. Rarely, major ischemic vascular disease of the leg may result in distal nerve damage and pain.

Some inherited conditions may be associated with painful distal neuropathy. Various infections infiltrate nerve and may cause a painful neuropathy. One of the most common is herpes zoster (i.e. shingles) that presents with pain and rash in a radicular pattern. After the rash has resolved, a significant number of patients are left with disabling neuropathic pain (postherpetic neuralgia). Lastly, amyloidosis is frequently associated with a small fiber painful neuropathy. Amyloidosis can occur as a familial disease or as an acquired condition. Amyloid deposits in nerve and may have a direct toxic effect or secondary vascular effect. The result is dysfunction of the small myelinated and unmyelinated axons. Patients typically present with painful polyneuropathy associated with loss of pain and temperature sensation and autonomic dysfunction.

The evaluation of a patient with suspected neuropathy involves first a close and detailed history noting the points above. EMG and nerve conduction studies are then required to confirm the localization is due to a polyneuropathy and not due to a plexopathy or polyradiculopathy. Second, the EMG and nerve conduction studies can often tell whether the neuropathy is primarily demyelinating or axonal. This is a key differentiating factor, as very few neuropathies present with primary demyelination. In some cases, a nerve biopsy is needed for definitive diagnosis. A nerve biopsy is usually required when inflammatory conditions such as vasculitis or infiltrative conditions such as amyloidosis are considered.

Therapy of neuropathic pain

The treatment of peripheral nerve disorders is divided into therapy of the underlying disorder and symptomatic therapy. When the etiology can be found, treatment of the underlying disorder is always preferable (e.g. B_{12} replacement for pernicious anemia with neuropathy, dialysis/transplantation for uremic neuropathies, immunosuppression for autoimmune inflammatory neuropathy, etc.). If the neuropathy is secondary to a toxic agent (e.g. alcohol), the first step is to prevent any further contact. In patients with entrapment neuropathy, surgical decompression may be useful in selected cases.

In cases where treatment for the underlying condition does not exist (i.e. inherited neuropathies) or the diagnosis is uncertain, symptomatic therapy must be employed (Table 7.3). Treatment of painful or other paresthesias is frequently difficult. Simple analgesics (ASA, non-steroidal anti-inflammatory drugs, acetaminophen) are usually tried first, but usually with no benefit. Narcotics are useful in selected cases, but are best avoided. Transcutaneous nerve stimulation and acupuncture are also useful in some patients.

Next employed are the agents which work directly on neuropathic pain. Among them are anticonvulsants (e.g. phenytoin, carbamazepine, neurontin, etc.), the tricyclic antidepressants (especially amitriptyline) and lioresal (baclofen). The agent of choice is usually based on the patient's other medical problems and their ability to tolerate potential side-effects. Amitriptyline is

Table 7.3 Therapy for neuropathic pain.

Analgesics
Transcutaneous electrical nerve stimulation
Tricyclic antidepressants
Anticonvulsants
Lioresal (baclofen)
Capsaicin ointment
Anti-arrhythmics
Biofeedback
Acupuncture
Neurosurgical ablative procedures
Multidisciplinary pain centers

among the most effective agents in the treatment of chronic neuropathic pain. However, several points must be kept in mind. First, mild anticholinergic side-effects (dry mouth, visual blurring, constipation) and sedation are dealt with by initially using a low dose (typically 10 or 25 mg) at bedtime. The dose can then slowly be titrated up to a more therapeutic level. It is not unusual that patients require 25–100 mg of amitriptyline at bedtime. Second, and more importantly, is the fact that the analgesic properties of amitriptyline are always delayed, usually several weeks. Patients need to be encouraged to stick with their program and not to give up too early. If the anticholinergic side-effects are too bothersome or contraindicated (e.g. urinary retention from prostatic enlargement), then other tricyclics with fewer anticholinergic side-effects (e.g. nortriptyline) can be substituted.

Other than the tricyclic antidepressants, the anticonvulsant medicines (e.g. phenytoin, carbamazepine, and neurontin) have antineuropathic pain qualities. Doses are similar to those used to treat seizures. In each, it is best to start at a low dose, and slowly titrate up to effect or until side-effects occur. Neurontin is particularly easy to use, not being associated with significant side-effects or drug interactions. Patients are usually started on a low dose (e.g. 100 mg tid) and slowly titrated up. Some patients may require total daily doses of 2400 mg or more.

In addition, lioresal (baclofen) has potent analgesic qualities. It is a first-line agent used in cases of trigeminal neuralgia, and is often helpful in neuropathic pain. Dosage is started at $^1/_2$ tablet (5 mg) tid and slowly increased by a $^1/_2$ tablet up to a maximum dose of 20 mg tid or qid.

The anti-arrhythmic, Mexitil (mexiletine), has been shown to be useful in some patients with diabetic polyneuropathy. This drug has significant potential toxicity (especially cardiac) and is best reserved for those familiar with its use and side-effects.

In addition to the oral medicines used to treat neuropathic pain, capsaicin ointment has been affective in some patients with neuropathic pain. It has been helpful in cases of postherpetic neuralgia, and diabetic polyneuropathy. Capsaicin suffers from the fact that it must be applied manually three or four times a day, and often causes increased symptoms during the first several days of therapy.

If patients cannot be managed with the above agents, they are best referred to a multidisciplinary pain center. Rarely, incapacitating neuropathic pain may require invasive, ablative neurosurgical procedures.

Of importance, many patients with neuropathic pain go through a phase where their neuropathy is quite painful. As the neuropathy gets worse, often their pain will get better. This occurs as frank numbness replaces painful paresthesias. Of course, numbness and lack of feeling may create a whole host of new problems. Among them, the most worrisome is injury to the foot without recognition, leading to more serious problems of infection of soft tissues and bone.

Suggested reading

Aids to the Examination of the Peripheral Nervous System. London: Baillière Tindall, 1986.

Al Hakim M, Katirji MB. Femoral mononeuropathy induced by the lithotomy position: a report of 5 cases and a review of the literature. *Muscle Nerve* 1993; **16**:891–895.

Bradley WG, Chad D, Verghese JP *et al.* Painful lumbosacral plexopathy with elevated erythrocyte sedimentation rate: a treatable inflammatory syndrome. *Ann Neurol* 1984; **15**:457–464.

Cimino WR. Tarsal tunnel syndrome: review of the literature. *Foot Ankle* 1990; **11**:47.

Katirji MB, Wilbourn AJ. Common peroneal mononeuropathy: a clinical and electrophysiologic study of 116 lesions. *Neurology* 1988; **38**:1723–1728.

Keck C. The tarsal tunnel syndrome. *J Bone Joint Surg* 1962; **44**:180.

Sander JE, Sharp FR. Lumbosacral plexus neuritis. *Neurology* 1981; **31**:470–473.

Schaumburg HH, Spencer PS, Thomas PK. *Disorders of Peripheral Nerves.* Philadelphia: F.A. Davis Co., 1983.

Wilbourn AJ. Radiculopathies. In: Brown WF, Bolton CF, eds. *Clinical Electromyography,* 2nd edn. Boston: Butterworth-Heinemann, 1993.

Yeun EC, Olney RK, So YT. Sciatic neuropathy: clinical and prognostic features in 73 patients. *Neurology* 1994; **44**:1669–1674.

CHAPTER 8

Other leg pain

Magruder C. Donaldson

A number of pain syndromes do not fit neatly into one of the foregoing chapters but are sufficiently common and troublesome to warrant discussion.

Abdominal and pelvic conditions

Abdominal and pelvic disease processes such as infection, hematoma and trauma may result in femoral neuropathy if the elements of the lumbar plexus (L2–L4) are directly affected. For example, contained rupture of an abdominal aortic aneurysm occasionally presents with pain in the distribution of the femoral nerve in the thigh. Another example of a pelvic condition causing leg pain is obturator hernia which occurs when a defect in the internal obturator fascia becomes sufficiently large to allow herniation of abdominal or pelvic contents into the obturator foramen. Incarceration or strangulation may result, with signs of inflammation or bowel obstruction. The diagnosis is often delayed because of the rarity of the condition. A mass may be evident in the medial thigh with the hip externally rotated and a pelvic mass may be apparent on rectal or vaginal examination (Figure 8.1). The Howship–Romberg sign may be elicited by external rotation of the hip causing pain radiating down the medial thigh in the distribution of the obturator nerve. Though somewhat controversial, the piriformis syndrome consists of sciatic neuropathy produced by impingement upon the sciatic nerve by the piriform muscle as both structures exit the greater sciatic foramen in the pelvis.

Soft tissue infection

Carbuncle, furuncle and cellulitis result from breakdown of the skin barrier. Diabetics are particularly susceptible, as are people with other conditions which affect the integrity of the skin. Chronic venous and arterial insufficiency are therefore often complicated by soft tissue infection. Seemingly trivial injury, insect bites or more substantial trauma all offer a portal for infection.

When contained to the skin and subcutaneous tissue, a carbuncle or furuncle is produced, most frequently by skin organisms such as *Staphylococcus aureus*. Localized swelling, redness and pain are typical, often maturing ('pointing') with spontaneous drainage. Lymphangitis may occur, classically with β-hemolytic streptococcus, even with a trivial initiating focus of infection. A

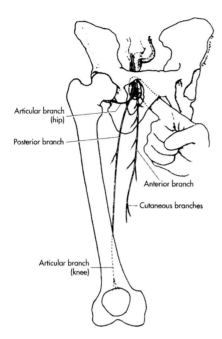

Articular branch
(hip)

Posterior branch

Anterior branch

Cutaneous branches

Articular branch
(knee)

Figure 8.1 Anatomy of obturator hernia, with protrusion of abdominal content into obturator foramen producing leg pain by impingement upon obturator nerve. Mass is often evident on rectal or vaginal examination. Reprinted with permission from Carter JE. Sciatic, obturator, and perineal hernias: a view from the gynecologist. In: Fitzgibbons RJ, Greenburg AG, eds. *Nyhus and Condon's Hernia*, 5th edn. Philadelphia: Lippincott, Williams & Wilkins, 2002, p. 544.

linear red streak is present from the portal of entry following the course of the lymphatics up the leg. Tender, swollen lymph nodes are evident in the groin or popliteal space and a high fever with systemic malaise are often present due to bacteremia. Cellulitis affects the subcutaneous tissues to a variable extent with induration, redness, swelling, and tenderness. A variety of organisms may be involved. Subfascial infection is very unusual without significant trauma or recent surgery, except in the foot. Classically in diabetics, a relatively innocuous appearing local portal of entry such as a plantar ulcer or paronychia gives rise to deep penetrating infection which ascends via the tendon sheaths into the joint spaces and deep structures of the foot and even into the ankle and calf. Necrosis of skin and deep tissue is common. Multiple organisms, including anaerobes such as *Bacteroides fragilis*, are often present working in synergy. Surgical drainage is usually an important adjunct to antibiotics in order to gain control of these infections.

On less frequent occasions, soft tissue infection results in necrotizing fasciitis or myonecrosis. These infections result in marked systemic response with fever and hemodynamic manifestations and local findings of progressive ecchymosis, bullae, dermal gangrene, edema and crepitus due to gas formation in the tissues. Although Gram-positive *Clostridia* species can produce gas gangrene, Gram-negative organisms such as *Escherichia coli* also produce gas in the tissues. These infections typically respond poorly to antibiotics alone and require urgent surgical debridement for control.

Differential diagnosis of soft tissue infection is mainly with superficial thrombophlebitis and other local inflammatory conditions such as gout and joint sepsis.

Muscle injuries

Forceful extension of the ankle may produce acute calf pain on the basis of musculotendinous strain or tear. Patients with plantaris muscle rupture usually have a suggestive history such as sudden onset of calf pain after stepping off a curb. Examination demonstrates tenderness in the calf exacerbated by ankle extension but with voluntary flexion intact, as opposed to complete Achilles tendon rupture in which flexion is lost. A similar traumatic history is consistent with painful tearing of muscles in the thigh. Hematoma results in an inflammatory reaction which adds to the pain syndrome. If encountered days after the injury, patients with rupture of thigh or calf muscles typically have ecchymosis at the ankle behind the medial malleolus from hematoma dissecting down the leg. Early ice, analgesics and rest are the cornerstones of management. Though the history is nearly pathognomonic for such injuries, either primary or secondary deep vein thrombosis and ruptured Baker's cyst must be kept in mind.

Chronic compartment syndrome

Chronic overuse or overconditioning of the legs, such as occurs with long distance running or other types of vigorous athletics, may result in recurring abnormally high fascial compartment pressure after onset of exercise. Pain occurs in the involved compartment at variable times after beginning repetitive muscle contraction with enough severity to compel cessation of exercise. Compartment pressure recedes with rest and the pain subsides. Evidence supporting the diagnosis may be obtained by correlating intracompartment pressure changes with symptoms during exercise on a treadmill. Therapy may require surgical fasciotomy if exercise moderation is not successful. Diagnosis involves exclusion of other entities, most importantly vascular disease causing arterial or venous claudication, and popliteal artery entrapment syndrome.

Causalgia

Causalgia, otherwise known as reflex sympathetic dystrophy and complex regional pain syndrome (see Chapter 2), is a disabling pain syndrome which occurs after trauma to the limb. The injury may be relatively slight, but more typically involves significant fracture or soft tissue damage involving surgery and immobilization. Though post-traumatic neuralgia, neuroma and neuropathy occur as a direct result of injury to the nerves themselves, causalgia is distinguished by the absence of motor or sensory deficits in the symptomatic portion of the extremity. Pain does not follow a clear anatomic dermatome and is generally constant with episodic exacerbation for no apparent reason. There are frequently accompanying vasomotor findings such as coolness and pallor. Sweating may occur as another manifestation of increased efferent sympathetic nerve activity. With chronicity, the muscles of the limb atrophy from disuse and the joints become stiff and even frozen. These late consequences may be sufficiently severe to become irreversible. Early diagnosis is critical to management, and relies on clinical presentation and trial temporary sympathetic blockade for confirmation.

Phantom pain

Phantom pain is a subjective complaint which occurs in mild form in a majority of patients early after major limb amputation. It persists at a significantly disabling level in no more than 10% of such patients. Patients report sensations which give the impression that the amputated limb is still present. The sensations are unpleasant and disquieting and may be interpreted as pain, particularly if the limb had been chronically painful prior to amputation. Symptoms tend to subside with time, and neurotropic medications may be helpful. Differential includes neuroma at the amputation site, usually evident on tapping the surgical stump for a Tinel's sign on physical examination.

Night cramps

Spontaneous muscular cramps occur in many people, and are frequently encountered in relatively elderly and less active individuals who present with multiple other causes of lower limb pain. Such cramps are common at night, interrupting sleep, and most often involve the muscles of the calves and feet. Patients on diuretics are more commonly afflicted. The cramps may be sporadic and unpredictable or chronically recurrent every night. They can be very painful, recede within a few minutes but frequently promptly recur. With familiarity, patients can feel a cramp coming on and may be able to ablate it by standing or massaging to stretch or relax the muscle. Prophylactic stretching of the ankles before bed can help reduce the incidence of cramps. Alternatively, quinine sulfate at bedtime is generally effective in preventing cramp attacks.

A related complaint has been called the restless leg syndrome. This benign condition involves an inability to find a comfortable and relaxed position for the limbs at night while trying to fall asleep. Patients describe dull aching, burning, drawing or numbness sensations, often bilateral, relieved by moving the legs. The condition can be sufficiently distracting to cause disabling insomnia, both in the patient and his bedmate. The cause is unknown, though there is an association with tension, stress and depression. Mild analgesics or tranquilizers at bedtime are typically effective in ablating the syndrome.

Suggested reading

Turnipseed W, Detmer DE, Girdley F. Chronic compartment syndrome: an unusual cause for claudication. *Ann Surg* 1989; **210**:557–564.

Weiner IH, Weiner HL. Nocturnal leg muscle cramps. *JAMA* 1980; **244**:2332–2333.

Young JR, Humphries AW, de Wolfe VG. Restless leg syndrome. *Geriatrics* 1969; **24**:167.

Appendix: Normal lower extremity anatomy

Figures in this section reprinted with permission from Agur AMR, Lee MJ. *Grant's Atlas of Anatomy*, 10th edn. Philadelphia: Lippincott, Williams & Wilkins, 1999.

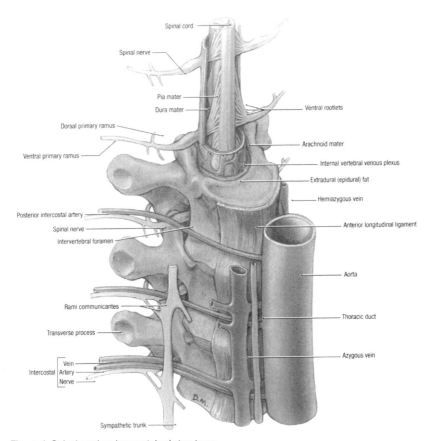

Figure 1 Spinal cord and prevertebral structures.

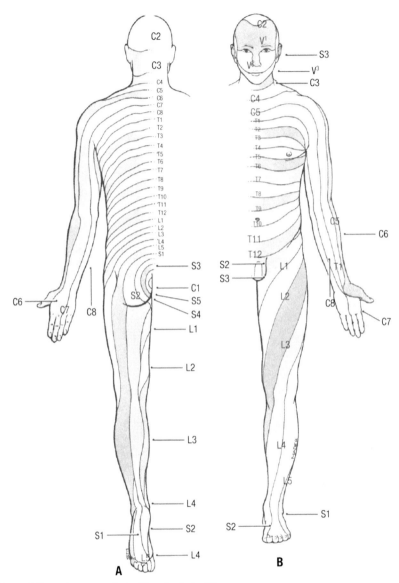

Figure 2 Dermatomes, posterior (A) and anterior (B).

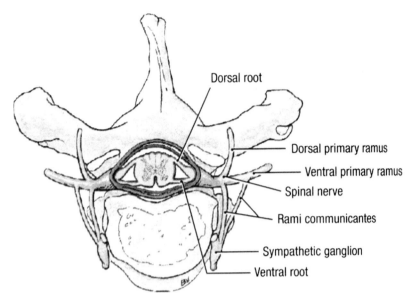

Figure 3 Formation of the spinal nerves.

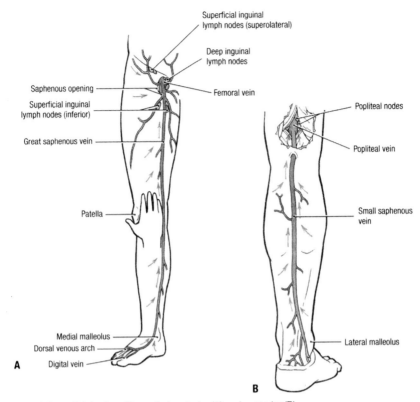

Figure 4 Superficial veins of lower limb anterior (A) and posterior (B).

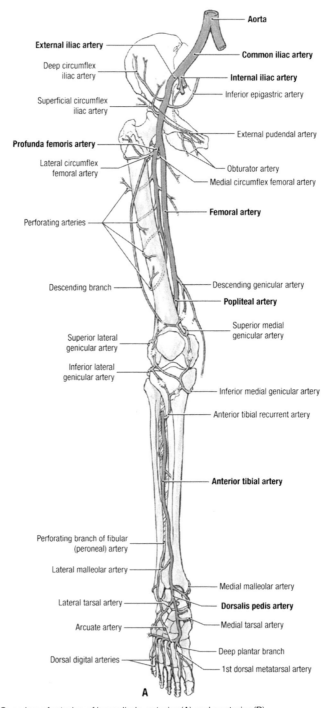

Figure 5 Overview of arteries of lower limb, anterior (A) and posterior (B).

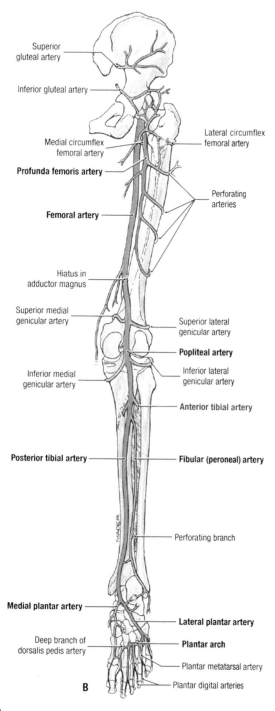

Superior gluteal artery

Inferior gluteal artery

Lateral circumflex femoral artery

Medial circumflex femoral artery

Profunda femoris artery

Perforating arteries

Femoral artery

Hiatus in adductor magnus

Superior medial genicular artery

Superior lateral genicular artery

Popliteal artery

Inferior medial genicular artery

Inferior lateral genicular artery

Anterior tibial artery

Posterior tibial artery

Fibular (peroneal) artery

Perforating branch

Medial plantar artery

Lateral plantar artery

Deep branch of dorsalis pedis artery

Plantar arch

Plantar metatarsal artery

Plantar digital arteries

B

Figure 5 (cont'd)

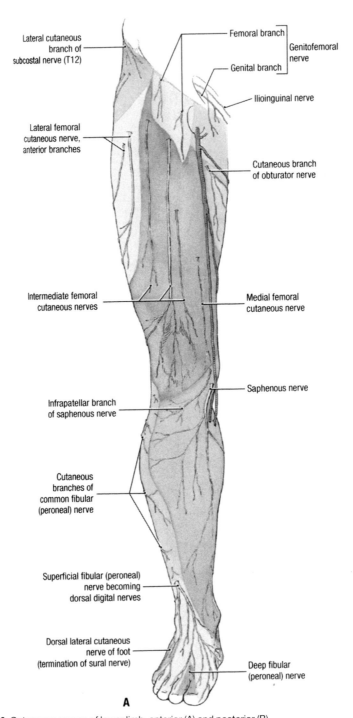

Figure 6 Cutaneous nerves of lower limb, anterior (A) and posterior (B).

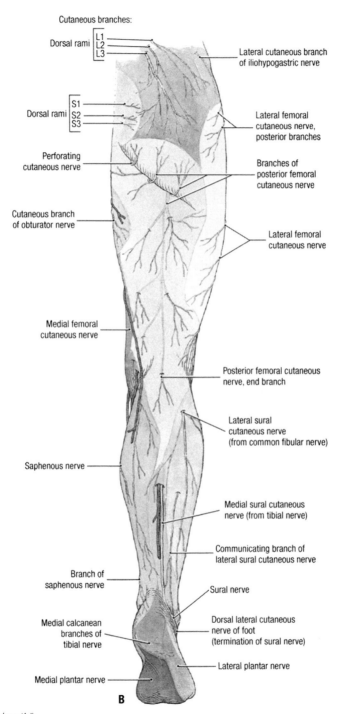

Cutaneous branches:

Dorsal rami L1
L2
L3

Lateral cutaneous branch
of iliohypogastric nerve

Dorsal rami S1
S2
S3

Lateral femoral
cutaneous nerve,
posterior branches

Perforating
cutaneous nerve

Branches of
posterior femoral
cutaneous nerve

Cutaneous branch
of obturator nerve

Lateral femoral
cutaneous nerve

Medial femoral
cutaneous nerve

Posterior femoral cutaneous
nerve, end branch

Lateral sural
cutaneous nerve
(from common fibular nerve)

Saphenous nerve

Medial sural cutaneous
nerve (from tibial nerve)

Communicating branch of
lateral sural cutaneous nerve

Branch of
saphenous nerve

Sural nerve

Medial calcanean
branches of
tibial nerve

Dorsal lateral cutaneous
nerve of foot
(termination of sural nerve)

Lateral plantar nerve

Medial plantar nerve

B

Figure 6 (cont'd)

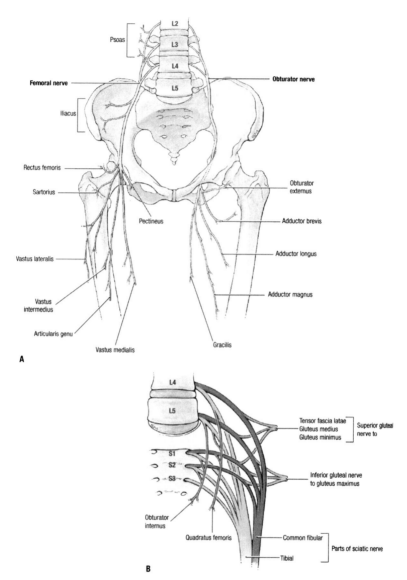

Figure 7 Overview of the motor distribution of lumbar (A) and sacral (B) plexus.

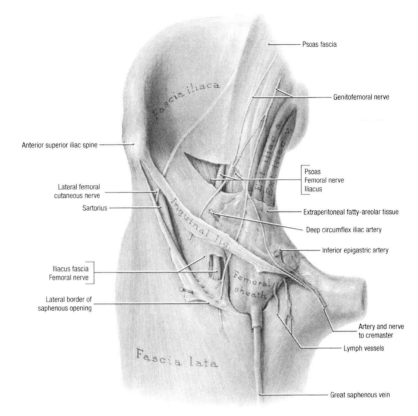

Figure 8 Femoral sheath.

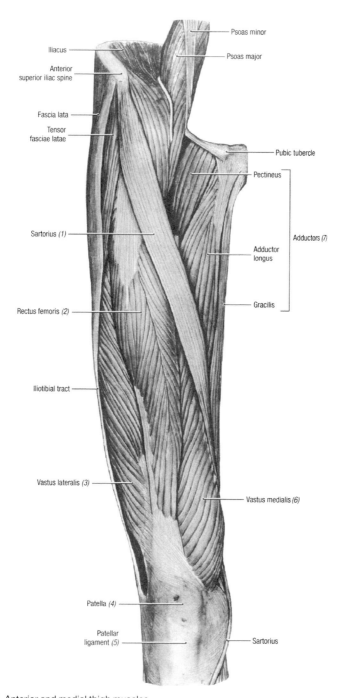

Figure 9 Anterior and medial thigh muscles.

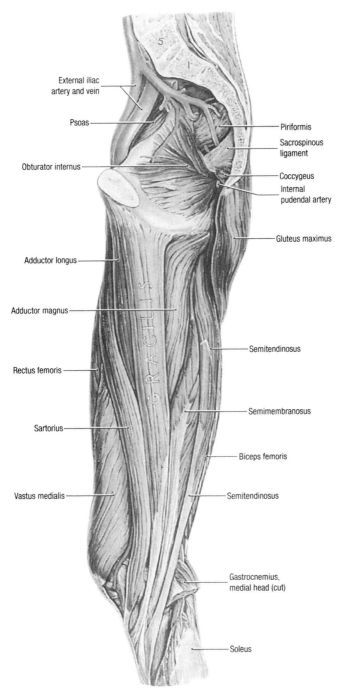

Figure 10 Muscles of medial aspect of thigh.

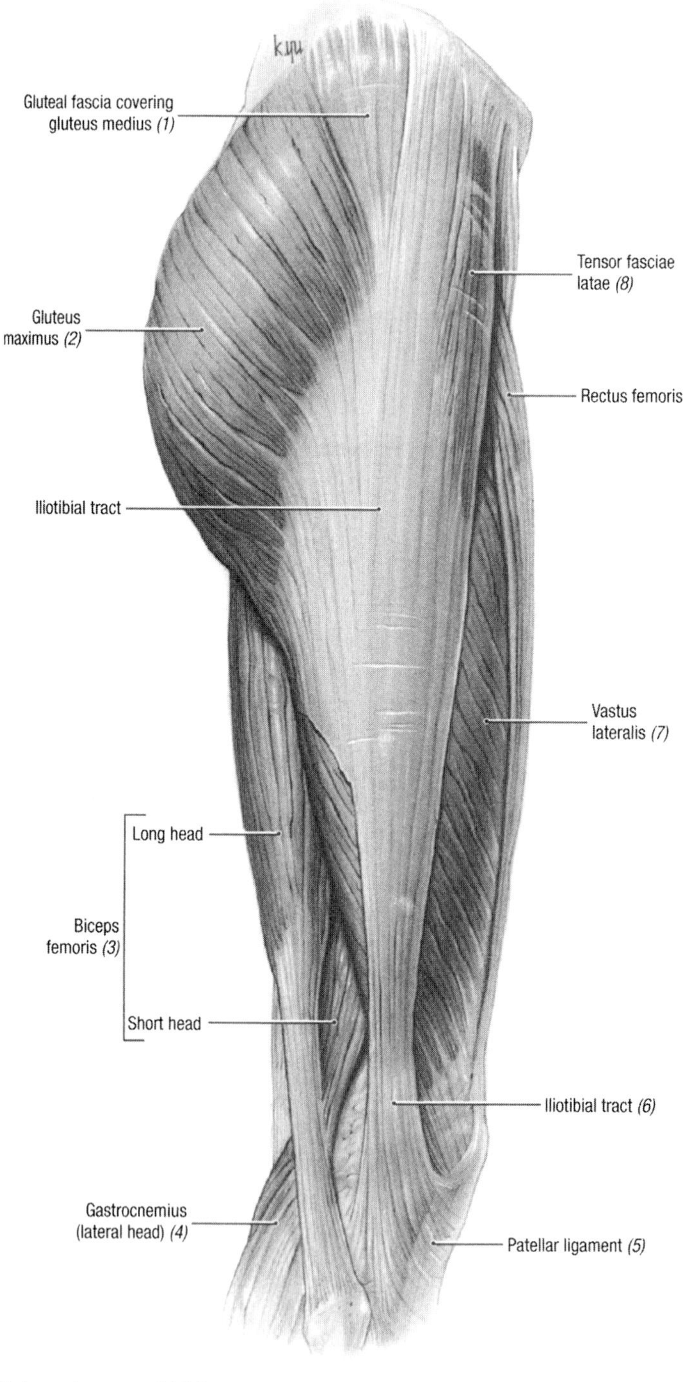

Gluteal fascia covering
gluteus medius (1)

Gluteus
maximus (2)

Iliotibial tract

Tensor fasciae
latae (8)

Rectus femoris

Vastus
lateralis (7)

Long head

Biceps
femoris (3)

Short head

Iliotibial tract (6)

Gastrocnemius
(lateral head) (4)

Patellar ligament (5)

Figure 11 Lateral aspect of thigh.

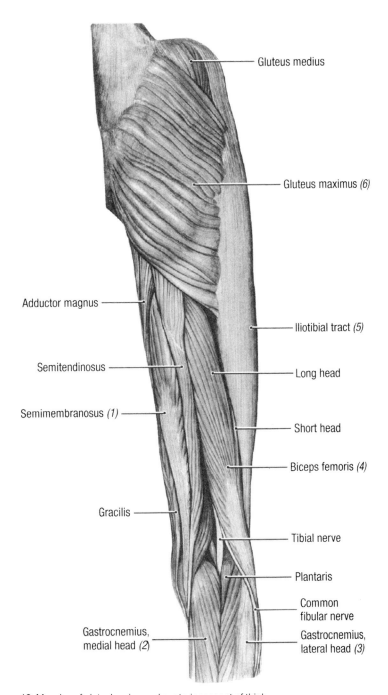

Figure 12 Muscles of gluteal region and posterior aspect of thigh.

SUPERIOR

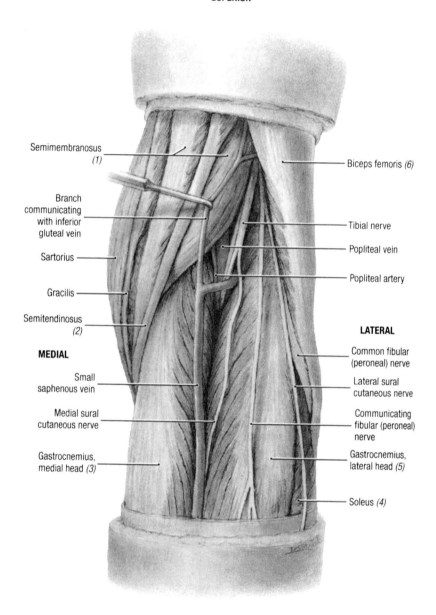

Semimembranosus *(1)*

Branch communicating with inferior gluteal vein

Sartorius

Gracilis

Semitendinosus *(2)*

MEDIAL

Small saphenous vein

Medial sural cutaneous nerve

Gastrocnemius, medial head *(3)*

Biceps femoris *(6)*

Tibial nerve

Popliteal vein

Popliteal artery

LATERAL

Common fibular (peroneal) nerve

Lateral sural cutaneous nerve

Communicating fibular (peroneal) nerve

Gastrocnemius, lateral head *(5)*

Soleus *(4)*

INFERIOR

Figure 13 Popliteal fossa, posterior view.

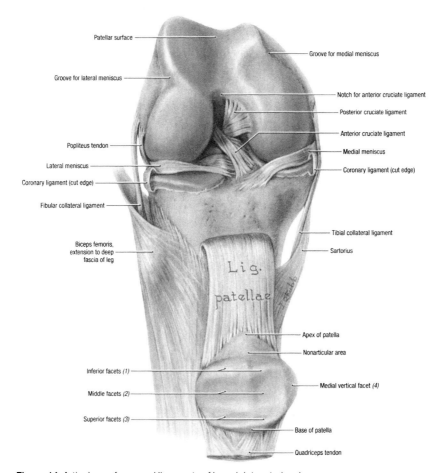

Figure 14 Articular surfaces and ligaments of knee joint, anterior view.

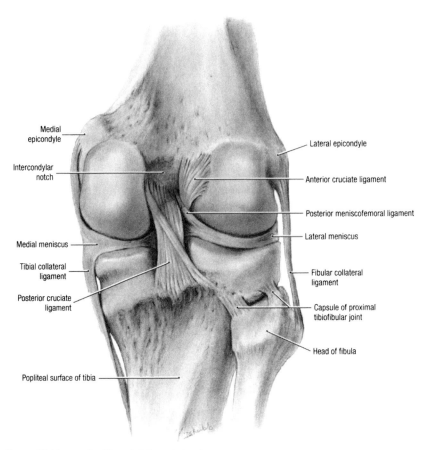

Figure 15 Ligaments of knee joint, posterior view.

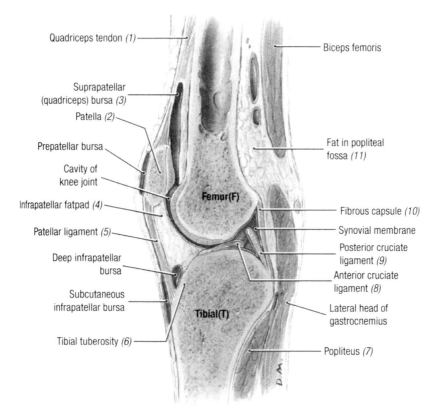

Quadriceps tendon *(1)*

Biceps femoris

Suprapatellar
(quadriceps) bursa *(3)*

Patella *(2)*

Prepatellar bursa

Cavity of
knee joint

Infrapatellar fatpad *(4)*

Patellar ligament *(5)*

Deep infrapatellar
bursa

Subcutaneous
infrapatellar bursa

Tibial tuberosity *(6)*

Fat in popliteal
fossa *(11)*

Femur(F)

Fibrous capsule *(10)*

Synovial membrane

Posterior cruciate
ligament *(9)*

Anterior cruciate
ligament *(8)*

Lateral head of
gastrocnemius

Tibial(T)

Popliteus *(7)*

Figure 16 Sagittal section of knee.

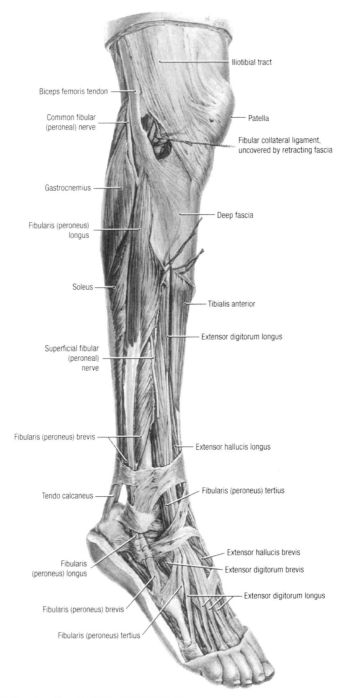

Figure 17 Muscles of leg and foot, anterolateral view.

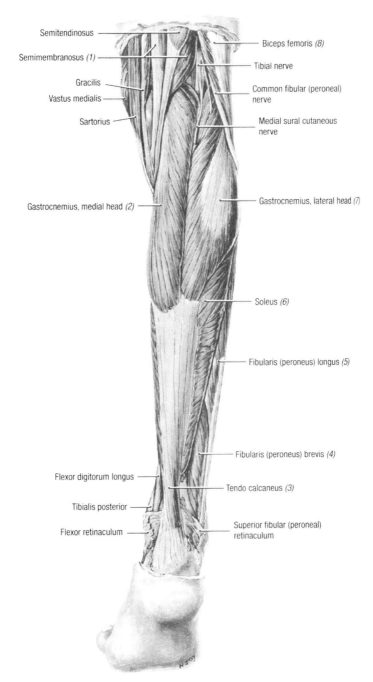

Semitendinosus

Semimembranosus *(1)*

Gracilis

Vastus medialis

Sartorius

Gastrocnemius, medial head *(2)*

Biceps femoris *(8)*

Tibial nerve

Common fibular (peroneal) nerve

Medial sural cutaneous nerve

Gastrocnemius, lateral head *(7)*

Soleus *(6)*

Fibularis (peroneus) longus *(5)*

Fibularis (peroneus) brevis *(4)*

Tendo calcaneus *(3)*

Flexor digitorum longus

Tibialis posterior

Flexor retinaculum

Superior fibular (peroneal) retinaculum

Figure 18 Posterior leg, superficial compartment.

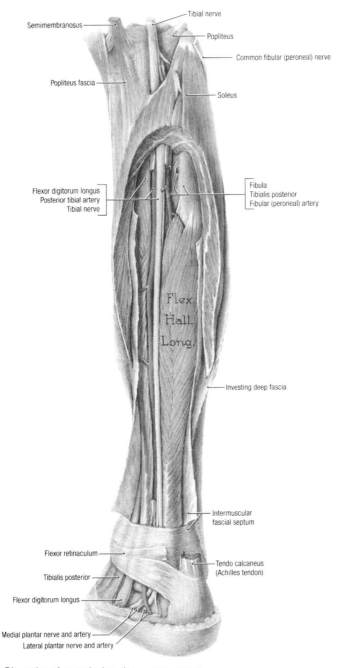

Semimembranosus

Tibial nerve

Popliteus

Common fibular (peroneal) nerve

Popliteus fascia

Soleus

Flexor digitorum longus
Posterior tibial artery
Tibial nerve

Fibula
Tibialis posterior
Fibular (peroneal) artery

Flex.
Hall.
Long.

Investing deep fascia

Intermuscular
fascial septum

Flexor retinaculum

Tibialis posterior

Flexor digitorum longus

Tendo calcaneus
(Achilles tendon)

Medial plantar nerve and artery
Lateral plantar nerve and artery

Figure 19 Dissection of posterior leg, deep compartment.

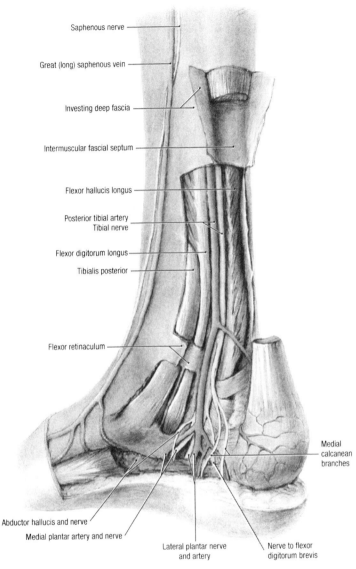

Saphenous nerve

Great (long) saphenous vein

Investing deep fascia

Intermuscular fascial septum

Flexor hallucis longus

Posterior tibial artery
Tibial nerve

Flexor digitorum longus

Tibialis posterior

Flexor retinaculum

Medial
calcanean
branches

Abductor hallucis and nerve
Medial plantar artery and nerve

Lateral plantar nerve
and artery

Nerve to flexor
digitorum brevis

Figure 20 Medial ankle.

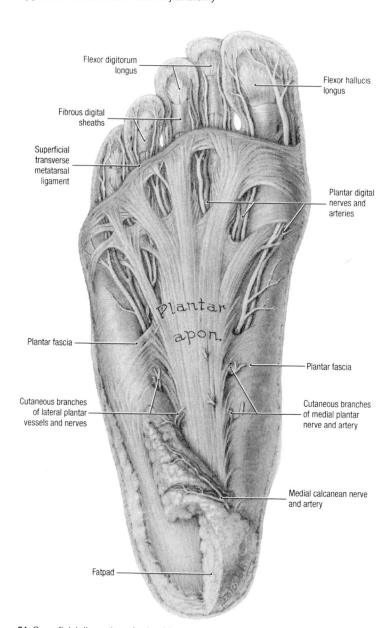

Figure 21 Superficial dissection of sole of foot.

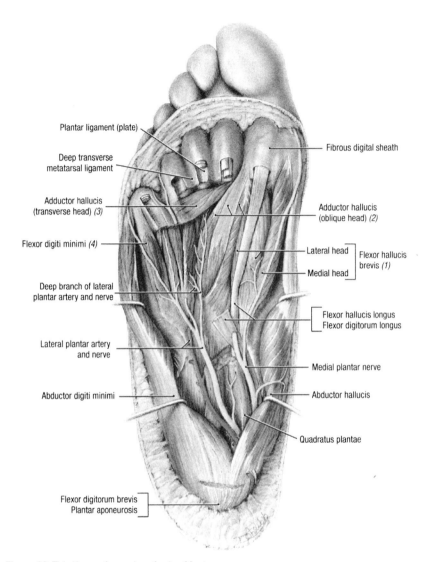

Plantar ligament (plate)

Deep transverse
metatarsal ligament

Adductor hallucis
(transverse head) *(3)*

Flexor digiti minimi *(4)*

Deep branch of lateral
plantar artery and nerve

Lateral plantar artery
and nerve

Abductor digiti minimi

Flexor digitorum brevis
Plantar aponeurosis

Fibrous digital sheath

Adductor hallucis
(oblique head) *(2)*

Lateral head
Medial head

Flexor hallucis
brevis *(1)*

Flexor hallucis longus
Flexor digitorum longus

Medial plantar nerve

Abductor hallucis

Quadratus plantae

Figure 22 Third layer of muscles of sole of foot.

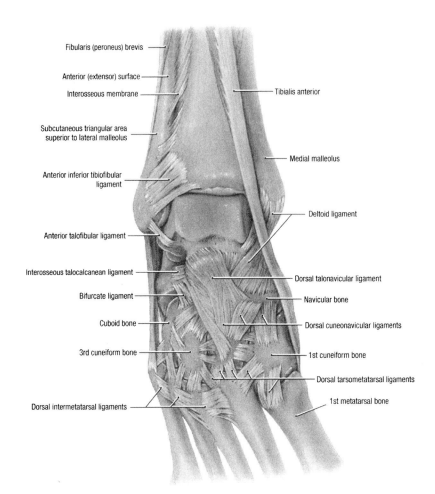

Fibularis (peroneus) brevis

Anterior (extensor) surface

Interosseous membrane

Subcutaneous triangular area
superior to lateral malleolus

Anterior inferior tibiofibular
ligament

Anterior talofibular ligament

Interosseous talocalcanean ligament

Bifurcate ligament

Cuboid bone

3rd cuneiform bone

Dorsal intermetatarsal ligaments

Tibialis anterior

Medial malleolus

Deltoid ligament

Dorsal talonavicular ligament

Navicular bone

Dorsal cuneonavicular ligaments

1st cuneiform bone

Dorsal tarsometatarsal ligaments

1st metatarsal bone

Figure 23 Ankle joint and joints of dorsum of foot.

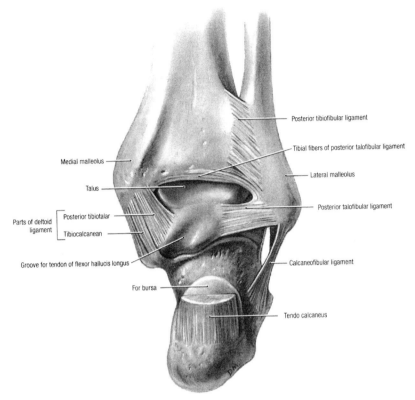

Figure 24 Ankle joint, posterior view.

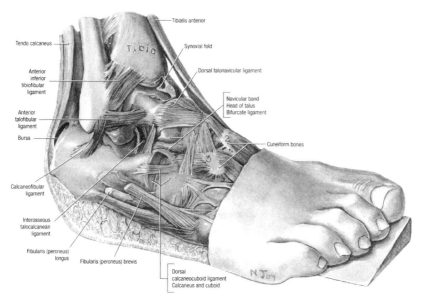

Figure 25 Joints of inversion and eversion.

Index

Notes: Page references in **bold** indicate tables or figures. Please also note that as the subject of this book, all entries refer to leg pain unless otherwise stated.